Living with Stroke

A Guide for Patients and Their Families

Fifth Edition
Richard C. Senelick, M.D.

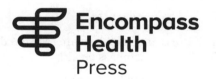

Encompass
Health
Press

This book is not intended to replace personal medical care and/or professional supervision; there is no substitute for the experience and information that your doctor or health professional can provide. Rather, it is our hope that this book will provide additional information to help people understand the nature of a stroke and its effects on those who are disabled and their families.

Proper treatment should always be tailored to the individual. If you read something in this book that seems to conflict with any of your doctors' or health professionals' instructions, contact them. There may be sound reasons for recommending a treatment or behavior that may differ from the information presented in this book.

If you have any questions about any treatment in this book, please consult your doctor or health care professional.

Also, the names and cases used in this book do not represent actual people, but are composite cases drawn from several sources.

This book is dedicated to the patients and families who live daily with the effects of stroke. For many, their lives have been changed permanently. They did not expect stroke to come to their houses, but, once it did, they adapted and developed strengths they never knew they had. They have learned there is life after stroke.

The Facts About Encompass Health

As a national leader in post-acute care, Encompass Health (NYSE: EHC) offers facility-based and home-based patient care through its network of inpatient rehabilitation hospitals, home health agencies and hospice agencies. With a national footprint that spans 127 hospitals and 237 home health & hospice locations in 36 states and Puerto Rico, the Company is committed to delivering high-quality, cost-effective care across the post-acute continuum. Driven by a set of shared values, Encompass Health is the result of the union between HealthSouth Corporation and Encompass Home Health & Hospice, and is ranked as one of Fortune's 100 Best Companies to Work For, as well as Modern Healthcare's Best Places to Work.

Some of its diverse services include the treatment of spinal cord injury, sports injuries, brain injury, stroke, pain management, oncology rehabilitation, geriatric rehabilitation and wound care.

Encompass Health Press has been created to help patients and their loved ones understand the implications of an injury or illness. All of its books are created to help them learn how to cope with life's unexpected changes. And, above all, each book is designed to show, in compassionate and intelligent terms, that you, the reader, are not alone.

Acknowledgments

I would like to recognize Encompass Health for its support of Encompass Health Press so that it can meet the educational needs of patients with disabilities and their families. The leadership of Mark Tarr has always made clear that the needs of patients and their families are a prime mission. A special thanks to Lisa Charbonneau, D.O. for her medical leadership, dedication to education, and guidance on numerous educational endeavors. Danny Kirkland, Joye Hansford and the entire production staff of Encompass Health Press provided limitless help and hours to the production of this and our other publications. To my wife Anne, whose understanding and independence allow me to be a complete physician and take on projects like Encompass Health Press.

Contents

It Will Never Happen to Me

It's one of our worst nightmares. It conjures up such fear that we may deny its possibility. We call it impossible and turn the other way.

Then again, perhaps we pray it will never happen—or that it can be taken away once someone we love is irrevocably changed. Whatever the array of emotions, the anger, the pain, the hopelessness, and the worry, when a stroke strikes a family member, one outcome is certain. Our lives will never be the same. Here are some sobering statistics:

- There are over 795,000 new and recurrent strokes each year.

- Someone in the United States has a stroke every 40 seconds.

- Stroke is the third leading cause of death in America today— and a leading cause of long-term adult disability.

- Approximately 160,000 people die from stroke every year—and 5.5 million survivors continue to suffer its aftermath.

- One out of every ten families is touched by stroke.

But there is good news. With proper care and knowledgeable rehabilitation, most stroke survivors can return home and resume their lives. As we hope to show within these pages, there is life after stroke.

A Woman's Tale

"My boutique had always done well. I carried classic styles, fashions that could easily be worn by teens and by my more mature customers alike. Dresses, suits, coats, accessories—even shoes and boots. I'd always done well and I loved my work. When my husband and I got divorced, I threw myself into my work more than ever. Today, I guess you could call me a working grandmother, but I don't like to admit to the grandmother part.

"When a nearby mall threatened to take away some of my business, I worked even harder, longer hours. Sundays. I wanted to keep my edge. One quiet afternoon, I was in the back, unpacking a new shipment of dresses. I'd picked up a garment—I remember it was a black sequined cocktail dress—and started to put it on a hanger when suddenly my left hand just stopped moving. There was this dress, half on a hanger. I was holding the hanger in my right hand; I dropped the dress. It was as if it had floated from my hand. I had no movement. No feeling. No sensation. The entire left side of my body felt heavy and numb.

"I yelled out. My voice sounded far away, as if I was talking on a bad telephone line. My mouth felt very dry; I couldn't move my lips very well. I yelled again, even though it sounded silly to me. I had to. My assistant was on the floor, helping a customer. She ran to the back and saw me standing in a pool of black sequins. I was gripping my desk with my right hand. If I had let go, I would have fallen. I had no control.

"It was the weirdest feeling. I had no pain, just numbness. Plus, I could think. I mean I knew who I was and I knew something was happening to me. I wasn't afraid, either, at least on one level. All I wanted to do was go home and go to sleep. I was very, very tired.

"Somewhere in my consciousness I knew I had just had a stroke."

This "working grandmother" was one of the lucky ones. She'd suffered a stroke, but it was only temporary. She listened to its warning, however, and worked on managing the stress in her life. She hired another person for the boutique. She went to her doctor for a complete evaluation, and she promised to see him for regular checkups. She started to take blood pressure medication every day without fail. She began an exercise program.

Within a few weeks, she was helping out at her grandson's birthday party. She had gone back to work on a part-time basis.

The fact is that not all strokes are horror stories. Like this woman's tale, they can have happy endings. But you must heed the signs. A stroke is not just an act of fate, a terrible quick brush with bad luck. Although its name might imply otherwise, a stroke does not happen in the blink of an eye.

It is the climax of a story that has been building for a long time, steadily working behind the scenes.

A stroke just doesn't happen overnight.

The Background Elements

The American Stroke Association's definition says it all: "A stroke occurs when blood flow to the brain is interrupted by a blocked or burst blood vessel."

Period. But this sudden disruption can be years in the making. It can be the result of clogged blood vessels in the brain, the buildup over time of the fatty cholesterol deposits that translate into atherosclerosis.

This disruption also can be created from a blood clot that travels to the brain from another part of the body, a clot that can become lodged in the blood vessels and, acting like a dam, stopping the blood supply from getting through to hungry cells.

Or, less commonly, a stroke can be caused by a weakness in blood vessel walls. This vulnerability, present from birth or from uncontrolled high blood pressure, eventually can cause a blowout in the vessel. The blood then will hemorrhage, or leak out, into the brain.

But whatever the disruption, the result is the same: the area beyond the clogged blood vessel, beyond the clot, beyond the hemorrhaging blowout, is not getting the blood supply that it needs. Like a lawn that isn't watered in a drought, this area of the brain begins to dry up, to shrivel. The brain cells that aren't "watered" will die very quickly.

And whatever function that area of the brain controlled will die also. This can be as basic a function as movement or swallowing—or as complex as the way the individual perceives the world or selects a piece of music.

Taking Stock

You can't change your birthright or your genes. Nor, in many cases, can you change the stressors that you have in your life, the pains or the losses. But you can do certain things to prevent a stroke, including

- getting your blood pressure measured at least twice a year—and taking your medication, if necessary, like clockwork

- watching your weight, eating sensibly, and exercising regularly

- having regular checkups to help catch stroke before it catches you. A doctor can tell you if your blood pressure is high, if your blood sugar is elevated, if your cholesterol levels are moving up, or if your heart is beating in an abnormal rhythm.

Furthermore, a doctor can help you recognize the most important indicator of all . . .

TIAs

TIA is a name to remember. It stands for transient ischemic attack and it can save your life. Sudden blurred vision, numbness or weakness, or difficulty in speaking that lasts only a few minutes or less than twenty-four hours can be a sign that things are amiss—and that it's time to take immediate care of yourself. In fact, if you experience these transient symptoms, you should call 911, immediately go to the emergency room, and hopefully prevent a stroke.

TIAs are one thing, however, and more debilitating strokes are another. For the latter, rehabilitation can mean the difference between dependency and independence, depression and acceptance, despair and hope.

When Someone You Love Has a Stroke

We have had a great deal of experience treating stroke. We have seen its debilitating results—but more often we have seen positive and successful outcomes. We have seen families torn apart by stroke—only to ultimately come together and adapt to their new roles.

We have seen, firsthand, in patient after patient, the results of successful rehabilitation.

We have seen that success in action.

We have seen hope become a reality.

But for those people who develop a stroke, for those living with a person who is suddenly different, that hope may be difficult to imagine.

Living with Stroke: A Guide for Families will help you determine how probable that hope is. It will help you cope with the aftermath of stroke.

Reading This Sourcebook

The first part of *Living with Stroke* is all about understanding. We will discuss, in depth, exactly what stroke is, the different types, the causes, and the risk factors. We hope that we can help you stop a stroke from happening—or stop it from recurring.

The second half of this sourcebook details the symptoms that can crop up when a stroke strikes. You also will discover the diagnostic tools that are used to determine a treatment plan.

The third section of *Living with Stroke* involves rehabilitation—the physical, behavioral, and cognitive treatments that work, that will help a stroke patient regain a life, whether it is getting up and walking around or communicating and acting in clear and appropriate ways.

Here, too, you will discover which medications work for both prevention and treatment. You will learn what you can expect from a rehabilitation hospital and the degree of assistance that you can expect.

Finally, and most importantly, in the fourth part of this book, you will learn the family's role. You will learn how to cope with your own overwhelming emotions. As you might already know, strokes do not affect just a single person. They happen to the entire family.

Focusing on you and on the rest of your family, this section also outlines the various problems that can crop up when a patient is ready to return home—from therapy noncompliance to a loss of sexual feeling, from anger and depression to adapting to a new career, from simply getting dressed in the morning to setting up the house to make it as accessible as possible.

And throughout all these pages, you will find words of inspiration, insights, research, ideas, and facts to help you keep going—and stay strong.

A Guide for Families

Family support is crucial. We have found that a good support structure—from a spouse, a family member, a circle of friends, a significant other—is vital to recovery.

Getting back does not happen in isolation.

There is life after stroke, but you must lend a helping hand.

Before we begin our medical journey, listen to these inspiring words from Helen Keller:

> "We could never learn to be brave and patient, if there were only joy in the world."

There is more than hope after the "dreaded impossible" happens. There is life.

PART I

A
Gathering
Storm

CHAPTER 1

Heart and Soul: Understanding the Brain and Heart Connection

"I never gave much thought to my body. It did what it was supposed to . . . until my stroke."

—*Sam, a sixty-two-year-old banker*

Stroke affects people in different ways. Sometimes there is a numbness, a tingling, an inability to speak, or an abrupt dizziness, as the following examples show.

- It was early. The rest of the family was asleep. Hal peered into the bathroom mirror. He touched his beard and made a face. He opened the medicine cabinet, took out his shaver, and, without warning, dropped it on the ground. Hal couldn't move his right hand. He couldn't bend down to pick it up. He started to yell, but his voice felt like cotton . . .

- Allison had had a terrible nightmare. The sky was dark; it was filled with swirling, spinning clouds. She was trying to walk through the cloudy landscape, but the fog, the moisture, and the wind were stopping her. The clouds were encircling her, choking her. Allison's eyes opened; she jolted awake. But the nightmare had not left. She could not see; she could not speak . . .

- Bill was climbing up the stairs with his new VCR when the pain struck. It only lasted a moment. A burst of light. A sharp headache. A tingling in his fingers. For one moment, he couldn't breathe or swallow. And then, as suddenly as it happened, it lessened. Bill was left with a thick tongue, a bit afraid, but he was definitely alive . . .

- Louise had been looking forward to this trip for years. The four-hour train ride was a piece of cake. When she saw her old friend, they hugged. They cried. It had been a long, long time. But now, under the comforter of the living room sofa bed, Louise was afraid. She was trembling. She couldn't see very well—even when she turned on the lamp. She was confused; she didn't know where she was. Her left arm felt numb. Her neck hurt and she was developing a headache . . .

These four people are experiencing strokes, some more serious than others, that hit them without any warning, any expectation. Why did this happen? Why now?

To understand why people have a stroke, you first must understand how the body functions—and malfunctions. You have to understand its vital connections, especially between the brain, the heart, and the blood that flows between them.

Because strokes, by definition, occur in the brain, let's begin at the top.

Brain Storming

Whoever coined "There's more here than meets the eye" could very well have been a neurologist. Frankly, it's not much to look at. A brain looks like a well-used sponge.

But appearances lie. The brain is bursting with energy. It consists of billions of nerve cells called neurons. And these neurons are settled in specific locales that are responsible for everything from the way we eat to the food we like. And this so-called "sponge" can soak up so much information that nothing, not even the most sophisticated computer in the world, can compare to it. Nothing.

As with most things, organization, delegation, and record keeping are crucial factors in its success. Despite its lumpy appearance, the brain is very active and very well organized—and in touch with all its "employees."

The Adjunct Staff: The Peripheral Nervous System

Veins, arteries, and nerves—all are intertwined, all are intricately spread throughout our bodies. When we touch a hot plate with our fingers, when we step on a nail, when we bang into the corner of a table, when we sip an ice-cold glass of champagne, whenever our senses are involved, so is our peripheral nervous system, sending our sensations, or stimuli, to our brain for responses. In normal brain functioning, the brain sends messages back down to those nerve endings, telling us to move our fingers from the hot plate or feel the pain of the nail, the table corner, the ice-cold ache of sipping a drink. The peripheral nervous system is like a vast messenger service, the adjunct staff so important to any successful organization.

But without the brain's interpretation, our sensations would mean nothing. We would feel nothing. When a part of our brain malfunctions, through either an accident or a stroke, we can lose the ability to identify, understand, and feel our sensations. They may become meaningless.

The Corporate Entrance: The Central Nervous System

The central nervous system (CNS) is like the North Star. It is the central operational system, or "office," where the peripheral nervous system, traveling from our fingers, our toes, our muscles, ends up. Specifically, the CNS consists of the spinal cord and the brain.

Secretarial Staff: The Brain Stem

This is the first stop in "the office." Because the brain stem resembles the brain of our cold-blooded friends, evolving more than 500 million years ago, it often is called the "reptilian" brain. And for snakes, lizards, and the like, this is as good as it gets. But for humans, the brain stem is only part of the whole—albeit a major part: it is vital for basic life-sustaining functions. Here, moving up from the spinal cord, you'll find the following:

The **medulla**—it doesn't get more life sustaining than this. The medulla is responsible for blood pressure, heart rate, even breathing in and out.

The **pons** is a type of bridge, connecting the medulla to the rest of the brain. But it doesn't just sit there, collecting tolls. The pons is home to the reticular formation, a mass of nerve fibers responsible for muscle tone, reflex actions, and alertness.

The **midbrain** is exactly that, a midpoint between the higher-functioning areas of the brain and the "reptilian" parts. Here, too, are more reticular formation functions, including eye muscle control and alertness.

Some Brain Facts

- The brain weighs almost three pounds.
- The brain is approximately the same size as a large cantaloupe.
- The brain consists of about 100 billion nerve cells.
- The number of ways that these nerve cells can be connected to each other is greater than the number of atoms in the entire universe.

The Office Coordinator: The Cerebellum

Just behind the brain stem, and slightly above it, sits the cerebellum, a mass of tissue that coordinates our every movement. It helps us keep our balance, allowing us to hold a glass of water steady. The cerebellum also coordinates the movements of our speech muscles.

Working with the cerebellum are the **basal ganglia,** located in the higher parts of the brain, helping to smooth the way we move. Obviously, a stroke in either of these two areas of the brain can affect our balance and our movements.

The Executive Assistant: The Diencephalon

This locale of the brain is the gateway to the higher-functioning areas of the brain. Situated right above the brain stem, the diencephalon is home to two crucial vice presidents.

The **thalamus** is a relay station that sorts out the messages traveling to the brain and decides which areas get what. It might send a message to several areas of the brain at once. When you step on a nail, for example, the pain will shoot through your brain stem to your thalamus and on to your memory storage bank. You might remember when you were a kid and had to get a tetanus shot because you stepped on a rusty nail. You might activate your thought processes, realizing that it isn't smart to walk around

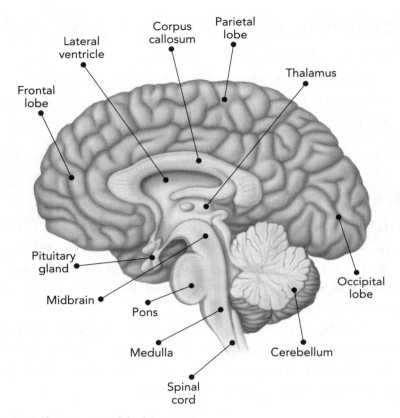

The different parts of the brain.

without shoes. The thalamus might bounce thoughts back and forth between those of your more curious, youthful days, your physical pain, and your fear of perhaps needing another shot.

The **hypothalamus** sounds like a relative—and it is. Although it's quite small, it wields much influence. Appetite control; sexual arousal; feelings of thirst, of sleep, of excitement; body temperature regulations; hormonal balance—the hypothalamus handles these and more, including a role in regulating moods and emotions.

The Executive Vice President: The Limbic System

Nowhere is the link between the parts of the brain more inter-related than that of thought and emotion. Pain, anger, joy, ela-tion—none of these would signify anything without linking them to our thoughts. The limbic system, a structure of interlocking nerve cells that lies between the diencephalon and the part of the brain that governs intellect, enables us to feel and express our emotions. You can feel the pain of that summer day when you were exploring by the sea, when you stepped on that rusty nail. You can remember the loneliness you felt at the resort's clinic, with its antiseptic walls and its kindly nurse. You can even feel embarrassed that you did it again as an adult, that you actually stepped on a nail because you were barefoot—even though you'd just told your child to put on his shoes.

The Boss: The Cerebrum

At last, the higher-functioning areas of the brain that separate us from lower animals. Here are our thoughts, our memories, our perceptions; and, like a presidential cabinet, it's divided into sev-eral separate, but equally important, areas.

The **amygdala** and the **hippocampus** take care of our thoughts and our memories. They give meaning to our emotions; they connect our thoughts, our senses, to the past. They are re-sponsible for the layers of memory, thought, and emotion that occur when, as adults, we step on that nail.

The **cerebrum** is the chunky brain stuff, the gray and white matter that makes up the majority of our brain. Covering it like an outer shell are layers of nerve cells, more gray matter, called the **cortex.** This part of the brain is responsible for our ability to move an arm or leg and to feel the different sensations. In short, here is where we learn, how we walk, how we understand, how

Adjoining Rooms

New studies have found that memory is not simply stored in one place. When a sensation is perceived, the hippocampus is responsible for retrieving various memories from different areas of the brain. The memory of a particular emotion, the ability to move in a specific way, the link back to other times—all these are collected and carried to the hippocampus through relaying neurotransmitters in the brain. The nearby amygdala gives these memories their emotional impact, their color, and their magic.

we communicate. Here is what, indeed, makes us human: the ability to form relationships, plan our future, and solve complex problems. A stroke in this area of the brain can affect our speech, our memory, our personality, our sensations, and our strength.

The Interoffice Network: The Right and Left Hemispheres

Look in the mirror. Imagine a line going straight down the middle of your head, dividing it into two perfectly similar mirror images. Indeed, it's as if there were a line dividing your brain into perfect halves. We call these exact replicas the right and left hemispheres of the brain. Despite the use of "right brain–left brain speak" by pop psychologists to help people find everything from their "inner selves" to great relationships, there are very real—and different—functions for each hemisphere.

The **corpus callosum** is a bridge, rich in nerve fibers, that connects the two halves of the brain, the right and left hemispheres.

The **left hemisphere** is most responsible for language, for speech and word usage. It is also the part of the brain most involved in reading, calculating, writing, and other forms of communication. It is responsible for movement and sensation on the right side of the body.

Location! Location! Location!

Ask any realtor and he or she will tell you: location is everything.

And that includes stroke. In fact, location is its most important characteristic.

Always remember: where a stroke occurs is much more important than how big it is.

The **right hemisphere,** on the other hand, gives language its color. It controls your visual memories, your "artistic" abilities to draw, dance, or play music. It is also responsible for your ability to see the bigger, long-range picture—as well as movement and sensation on the left side of the body.

But both hemispheres are needed to complete a whole. You might be able to speak if your left hemisphere is intact, but your right side gives that speech its rhythm, its inflection, and its personal texture and dash.

When a stroke occurs in one hemisphere, the opposite side of the body will be affected. In other words, if the left hemisphere of your brain is injured, the right side of your body might be paralyzed or weakened, and vice versa.

There are also different emotional symptoms. A left-hemisphere stroke can cause depression, but a stroke in the right hemisphere might create complete denial of the illness. (We'll be discussing all the different symptoms in both right- and left-hemisphere strokes in later chapters.)

Branch Offices: The Lobes of the Brain

Yes, it's true that your brain has specific locales that are responsible for different brain functions. It's also true that your brain is divided down the middle, into two separate, but equal, halves. But there's more. Each half has four lobes, each with different

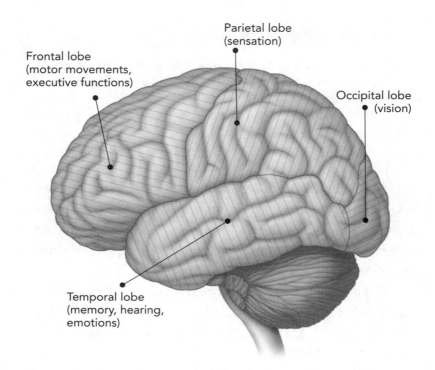

Parietal lobe
(sensation)

Frontal lobe
(motor movements,
executive functions)

Occipital lobe
(vision)

Temporal lobe
(memory, hearing,
emotions)

The lobes of the brain.

functions, each affecting you in different ways if a stroke happens to strike.

The **frontal lobes** could be considered the chief executive officers of the brain because they control so much of who we are: impulses, motivation, social interaction, communication, and voluntary movement. The "motor strip" that is responsible for all movement on the opposite side of the body is located in the frontal lobes—which are also responsible for our "executive functions": our ability to plan and to organize, to concentrate and to make decisions, to set goals, and even our capability to retrieve memory from storage. They are, as the name implies, in the front of the brain, and a stroke here could make a person incapable of saying what she means. It could make her agitated and impulsive. It might "flatten" her emotions, making her unable to generate new thoughts or plans. She might lose the ability to move all or part of the opposite side of her body.

The **temporal lobes** are our "temples" to memory. They hold our remembrances of both recent and distant pasts; they hold our learned fund of knowledge and information. Furthermore, the temporal lobes affect our emotional thought as well as our ability to hear and to appreciate music; they process the perceptions that flood the brain, making sense of our world. Located just behind and just below the frontal lobes, they also are crucial for who and what we are. A stroke here could make a person forget what he just said. It could make him unable to remember how to perform a task he has done a thousand times before.

The **parietal lobes** are very "sensitive." Situated just above the ears and in the back half of the brain, they are responsible for our sense of touch. They also are necessary when it comes to academics. They help us understand what we read and where things are in space. A stroke here can impair a person's ability to recognize an object. It can prevent her from comprehending the words she reads. She could feel numbness on the opposite side of her body. She could be unable to identify objects placed in her hand.

The **occipital lobes** control our vision. They are literally "the eyes in the back of your head." A stroke here can cause blindness or loss of a part of a person's vision. He might lose the ability to see the left side of his world if the stroke was in the right occipital lobe.

But the sites and arenas of brain function are only part of the picture. As with all relationships in life, communication is key. The different areas of the brain and the central nervous system itself must "speak" to each other. Messages must be relayed.

Whether it is stepping on that rusty nail, understanding the words in *War and Peace,* or simply breathing in and out, the brain must receive information—and send out a response.

Communication Network

Messages are relayed throughout the brain by a network of brain cells, **neurons,** and the "cables" that connect them: **axons.** The messages travel by both electrical impulses and by the release of chemicals called **neurotransmitters.**

Let's say you step on that ubiquitous nail. The "ouch!" of pain travels up the nerves from your foot, moving merrily along the axon. Suddenly, it reaches a space at its next stop in the spinal cord. This space is called a **synapse.** The next neuron lies in wait, but the electrical version of the message "ouch!" cannot reach it—at least not yet.

But the body is a master of problem solving. That same electrical charge that carried "ouch!" along the axon now triggers the release of a chemical: the neurotransmitter. This neurotransmitter crosses the synapse space to a **receptor,** waiting and ready, on the next cell. As soon as the chemical-conducted "ouch!" touches the receptor, it turns back into an electrical impulse and the message "ouch!" continues on its way toward the brain.

This process continues throughout the nervous system, through every area of the brain, at a fast and furious pace: countless messages bouncing back and forth, commands being shouted, information being stored, perceptions being understood, millions and millions of messages perfectly relayed in less than a second, every hour of the day.

Even more fascinating is the fact that chemical neurotransmitters know what electrical charge will trigger them. They will be triggered by only one "Mr. or Ms. Right." The electrical charge

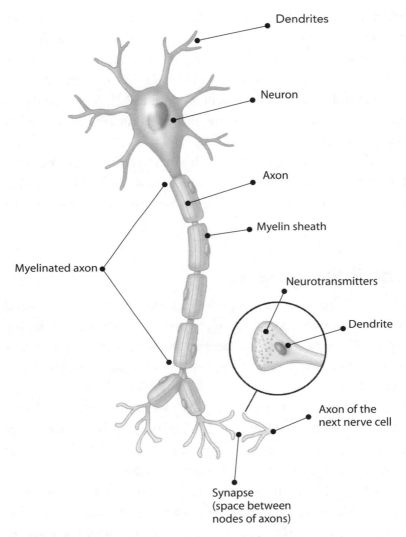

Dendrites

Neuron

Axon

Myelin sheath

Myelinated axon

Neurotransmitters

Dendrite

Axon of the
next nerve cell

Synapse
(space between
nodes of axons)

A neuron, complete with axon, dendrites, and synapses.

must match up with a specific chemical for the message to jump
the synapses. Without the right message, a chemical neurotransmitter will not be triggered. It will lie dormant, silent, quiet.

This is all well and good when the brain is functioning normally, when specific messages are being relayed. Unfortunately,

when a stroke strikes, some of the brain cells and axons can be damaged and messages just won't get through. Damaged synapses and neurons can create imbalances, affecting mood, emotions, and thought. A stroke in the temporal lobe can affect the connections there, preventing memory retrieval. A damaged synapse in the right hemisphere might prevent movement on the left side of the body.

Yes, strokes take place in the brain, but their beginnings may start far away and travel to the brain—via a clot in the blood that is pumped, filtered, and carried to and from the brain via the heart.

The Pulsing Heart

The brain feeds on oxygen, which is extracted from red blood cells. It's assured a constant supply from the high-speed pumping action of the heart, which, despite the soul-searching words of poets and philosophers, is actually a "hard-body" muscle that is about the size of a fist.

This "fist," however, can squirt a jet of life-sustaining blood several feet. You can feel this jet of blood surging through your body by taking your pulse. Each beat of your pulse pushes out about one cup of blood into your bloodstream.

But quality is more important than quantity. Believe it or not, our bodies contain only about twelve pints—or twenty-four cups—of blood. This is equivalent to approximately six quarts of milk or the weight of one Thanksgiving turkey.

However, these twelve pints pack a mighty wallop.

The Ultimate Recycling Machine

The twelve pints of blood pumped by the heart are, in effect, used over and over again. They go around and around in an endless circle throughout our bodies, delivering the blood's oxygen to all our organs and taking away their wastes.

This process is called circulation. Briefly, here's how it works:

1.   The heart is divided into four chambers, the right and left atrium and the right and left ventricle. The oxygen-filled blood from the lungs comes into the **left atrium** of the heart. It moves into the **left ventricle** and is pumped out into the bloodstream through . . .

2.   . . . the **aorta,** the "king" of all arteries. From the aorta, blood, carrying our body's fuel and food, travels through its passageways called **arteries.** The walls of the arteries are very elastic; they are muscular tubes that branch out, becoming smaller and smaller, until they are only one cell thick . . .

3.   . . . and fuel and oxygen can pass through them. These tiny arteries are called **capillaries.** The hungry cells in the body, from the muscles to the brain, from the kidneys to the liver, "eat" their fill and deposit carbon dioxide through their cell walls. The depleted, waste-carrying blood now begins its journey home through . . .

4.   . . . the **veins.** The blood is now more sluggish. The heart has used most of its energy to pump oxygen-rich blood into the body; it has less "oomph" for the return trip. Thus, the veins have little "pockets" or valves that catch any "back-flow" to make sure the blood keeps moving toward the heart

and doesn't get backed up. The veins get bigger and bigger until they reach the . . .

5.   . . . **right atrium** of the heart. As the heart pumps and clenches, this blood is pushed into the . . .

6.   . . . **right ventricle,** where it travels to the lungs and fills up once again with oxygen. This oxygen-rich blood journeys back to the left side of the heart, and the cycle begins anew.

The Blood's Push and Pull

Like the water in your house, circulation needs pressure to keep moving. Your blood pressure is what keeps your blood flowing and moving in a rhythmic way through your arteries.

When you get your blood pressure taken, the upper number in the reading, called the **systolic** pressure, reflects how hard your heart has to squeeze and contract to push the blood through your arteries. A high reading means that your heart is having to squeeze too hard to keep your blood moving.

The lower number, or the **diastolic** pressure, reflects the pressure in your arteries while the heart rests between beats. A high number here means that the pressure remains elevated even when your heart is resting between beats.

How Important Is Oxygen to the Brain?

Without it, the brain's entire electrochemical process will not work.

Without it, brain function in that oxygen-deprived locale will not take place.

Without it, we will lose consciousness within five to ten seconds.

Without it, we will experience brain damage within minutes.

Blood flow, its rhythm and pressure, can be affected by hereditary factors, kidney disease, weight gain, and cholesterol, a waxy substance that is carried through the bloodstream. As it builds up, cholesterol is deposited on the arterial walls. Eventually, the walls of the arteries thicken to the point where blood may not get through. If these deposits occur in the arteries feeding the heart, this can result in a heart attack. If they accumulate in the arteries feeding the brain, this can result in a stroke.

Because both high blood pressure and elevated cholesterol are important factors in stroke, we'll be discussing them, as well as the other risks, in more detail in the next chapter.

Food for the Brain

The brain has a hungry man's appetite. It needs 20 percent of the total blood supply to get the oxygen and food that it needs.

The crucial arteries through which the heart pumps blood up to the hungry brain are called the **carotid arteries.** Both the right and the left carotid arteries are all-important, branching out into a series of arteries in the front of the neck and into the brain. These arteries grow smaller and smaller as they travel, allowing all the areas of the brain, from the thalamus to the hippocampus, from the frontal to the temporal lobes, to get "served" with oxygen-rich blood.

But the carotid arteries do have a partner. Blood also travels to the brain through the **vertebral arteries.** These go up the vertebral column in the back of the neck, to form the basilar artery in the brain stem.

A stroke will have different symptoms if it occurs within the carotid system or within the areas of the brain fed by the vertebral arteries, and we'll be discussing these in more detail later.

We now have seen how the brain and the heart are connected. But before we close, let's briefly go over the chemistry of their common thread.

Life-Sustaining Fluids

Blood. We can be upset by the sight of it or donate it to save a life. But whatever the "gut feeling," blood is literally a carrier—of life. Think of it as a highly reputable moving van, a transporter that carries necessary food to our cells. And there is much more than meets the eye in its red color. If you put a drop of blood under a microscope, you'd see all of the following:

Plasma is the liquid that holds the blood cells; it gives the blood its consistency.

The **red blood cells** (or **corpuscles**) hold the food. They contain the oxygen and the other nutrients (in the chemical form of glucose) that the body needs to survive. After the various organs finish their "meal," these red blood cells head for the veins, carrying back the "empty plates" to the heart. Red blood cells also give the blood its red color.

The **white blood cells** are the "superheroes." They respond to "foreign invaders," both by fighting infection and by increasing in number when infection or inflammation threatens the body.

The **platelets** are responsible for clotting. When you cut yourself, platelets "rush in" and begin to create a web, a microscopic gauze of fiber, that traps other blood cells to stop the flow of blood.

Problems can arise, however, in the most well-oiled machine—and the human body is no exception. Clotting is crucial if you fall and hurt your knee, if you step on that ever-present nail. However, especially as we get older, our arteries can narrow and develop rough areas, which draw the attention of the platelets.

Pain in the Neck

The vertebral column in the neck is particularly vulnerable to bone spurs. These spurs can compress the arteries traveling through them and, consequently, may affect their blood supply.

Although not so serious as a stroke in the carotid system, these spurs may cause dizziness in elderly people, especially when they bend their heads back. Perhaps you, or someone you love, have experienced this phenomenon when getting a shampoo at a beauty salon. As you bend your head backward into the sink, you might experience some dizziness, which usually stops as soon as you sit up.

But, here, clotting is not so simple as a Band-Aid and a scab. Platelets don't always know when to stop their clotting action on these internal "cuts." Red blood cells soon will join in the fray; the clotting mass will get bigger and bigger. Passageways can become clogged, preventing blood from moving through the artery.

When this clotting takes place in the brain, it can result in stroke—and we'll be covering this phenomenon in more detail in Chapter 3.

Coming Together

Let's go back for a moment to that nail. There you are, on that hot summer day, walking barefoot on the sand. You step on that nail.

Pain immediately shoots up your nervous system to your brain, which sends out a response. "Ouch!" Your body goes into action. Your heart starts to pump a bit faster. You look down at the source of your pain and notice the blood on your foot. Clotting begins.

Other messages are sent: you remember the last time you stepped on a nail, that hot summer day when you were a child,

Some Blood Facts

- Blood is bright scarlet red in the arteries, but a deeper crimson in the veins.

- Blood is heavier than water but only by a small amount.

- The blood in men weighs more than the blood in women.

- Altitude affects our blood. Higher altitudes increase the amount of red blood cells in our system so that they can carry more oxygen.

when you'd been on a glorious vacation. Your memory is bitter-sweet and tinged with fear: you probably will need a tetanus shot. You admonish yourself: you should have been wearing shoes. You should have known better.

Your emotions affect your heart rate. Blood continues to surge. You might feel flushed.

And all these connections, all these responses, emotional, mental, and physical, occur in a fleeting moment of time.

This, then, is the heart, brain, and blood connection, a powerful triumvirate. As we have seen, all three play a critical role in our health—and in a possible stroke.

But there's more. The heart, the brain, and the blood are responding to something else. That's where the risk factors of stroke come in.

Risk Factors

"It was bad enough that my husband had
high blood pressure. But he was overweight,
he smoked, and he was a real couch potato
when he came home from work. When he
had a stroke, he was surprised. I wasn't."

—*Wife of a sixty-eight-year-old stroke patient*

Betty wasn't stupid. She knew that smoking was bad for her. She tried to stop several times, but she never made it past five months. Something always made her go back—stress, weight gain, boredom.

She didn't exercise either—although she did join the local Y and went to an aerobics class for a few weeks until some other event came up.

Betty hated her lifestyle, but instead of changing it, she plunged in and continued to spiral down. The more she fretted, the more she smoked—and ate. The more she smoked and ate, the more she fretted. It was a vicious cycle, with, she rationalized, no room or time left for exercise.

Yet Betty managed to beat the odds. She was a successful buyer in a major department store chain. She managed to raise her daughter alone after her husband died from an unexpected heart attack. She had a wide circle of friends and went out almost every Friday and Saturday night. She complained about her bad habits; she made jokes about them. But she didn't change them. And if the truth be known, she didn't think she really had to. She had yearly physicals and was always just fine, thank you.

Three weeks ago, Betty turned fifty. Three days later, she went for her physical, expecting to get her usual clean bill of health and lecture about her unhealthy lifestyle. But this time, her doctor looked serious. He wasn't smiling. He told her that she had diabetes and that her blood pressure was up. Not only did she have to go on medication, but she had to change her lifestyle immediately.

Betty had become a prime candidate for a stroke.

Risks are not engraved in stone. They don't mean certainty; they don't exclusively control fate. Instead, risks are what their name implies: greater odds.

If you continue on a specific route, in a specific lifestyle, you can be at risk if that lifestyle is a destructive one.

Some risk factors are greater than others. Some cannot be changed. But some, such as Betty's smoking and obesity, can be altered. Once the risk factor is treated, so is the risk. And the more risks that can be reduced, the healthier the remaining combination and the lower the risk across the board.

There are several risk factors in stroke. Some of them are the "luck of the draw," heredity, and time. But others are preventable and may be a question of bad habits—and within your control to change.

Knowledge is power. Recognizing these risk factors can help you reduce *their* power. To that end, let's go over them now.

Learn These Stroke Prevention Guidelines

1. Know your blood pressure and if it is elevated, get it treated.

2. If you are diabetic, tightly control your diabetes.

3. Find out if you have high cholesterol and treat it.

4. If you smoke, stop.

5. Include exercise in the activities you enjoy in your daily routine.

6. Adopt a healthy diet.

7. Find out if you have atrial fibrillation.

8. Control your weight—obesity kills.

9. If you drink alcohol, do so in moderation.

10. If you experience any stroke symptoms, seek immediate medical attention—call 911.

The Silent Killer—Hypertension

If there is one single highest risk factor in stroke, it is high blood pressure, or hypertension. A national survey found that between 40 percent and 70 percent of the people who had strokes also had high blood pressure. The groundbreaking Framingham study, which has followed more than 5,000 men and women for more than fifty years, continues to find that people with hypertension are two to four times more likely to have a stroke than those with normal pressure. And the Systolic Hypertension in Europe Study showed that even moderately high blood pressure can cause a stroke.

Although hypertension can be inherited, the reasons people get it are a mystery in the majority of all cases.

However, we do know *what* happens. As we have seen, the buildup of arterial pressure means the heart is working more— harder and faster. It also means that the small blood vessels are holding back the flow of blood, building up pressure behind them.

How Do You Know If You Have High Blood Pressure?

If your reading is greater than 140/90, you clearly have high blood pressure. However, in recent years it has become clear that people with "prehypertension," blood pressure greater than 120/80, will go on to develop hypertension and need treatment. You cannot ignore a little bit of high blood pressure—it may kill you!

Additional good news: medication works. If you have hypertension, your physician can prescribe a medication that works well for you.

But you must remember to take your medication exactly as your doctor prescribes and under her close supervision. The reason why hypertension medication doesn't always work is simple: people just stop taking it.

In addition, the blood vessels themselves are getting extra wear and tear and weakening to the point where a stroke is possible. And finally, high blood pressure can accelerate atherosclerosis, or hardening of the arteries, and increase the risk of heart disease, both of which are additional risk factors in stroke.

Yes, there is no doubt that hypertension is deadly. What makes it worse is the fact that there are no symptoms. It is completely silent, carrying on its destruction quietly over time, until the buildup of pressure and weakened artery walls result in a stroke.

In the past, people did not know they had hypertension until it was too late, until they had a stroke or a heart attack. Today, more and more adults are becoming savvy. They get their blood pressure checked at least annually. Indeed, studies have found that the successful treatment of hypertension can dramatically reduce the risk of stroke by more than 40 percent.

The White Coat Syndrome

Some people react to their doctor's presence with high blood pressure. Called the "White Coat Syndrome," this brief, momentary elevation of blood pressure is a normal reaction to the stress of waiting in an examination room for the doctor (in the white coat) to take a reading. If your blood pressure is initially high, your physician will most likely take another reading after ten or fifteen minutes. She might also suggest you monitor your blood pressure at home, with a kit you can purchase at the pharmacy. By taking your blood pressure over a period of weeks or months, you will get a more accurate reading.

The Age Factor

High blood pressure can be regulated. You are in control. But some of the risk factors of stroke are beyond your powers. They are simply a fact of life. Aging is one of them.

As you age, your arteries become more fragile. They are less elastic and flexible. They become brittle. This hardening of the arteries is called atherosclerosis. The more the buildup of atherosclerosis, the more likely these arteries are to clog or close off. If this occurs in the brain, it will result in stroke.

Diabetes Complications

At first glance, diabetes seemingly has nothing to do with stroke. After all, it is a disease that impairs the body's ability to control the level of sugar. But below the surface of that definition is a very strong—and dangerous—connection. Diabetes can affect circulation. And poor circulation can affect the blood vessels, especially the small capillaries in the eyes. Here, because of weakened, impaired blood vessels, diabetes can cause hemorrhages and blindness. Likewise, similar hemorrhages within the brain

A Reality Check

A sobering fact of life: two-thirds of all strokes occur in men and women over the age of sixty-five.

But the risk of stroke can be reduced whatever your age through a program of exercise, regular blood pressure readings, and routine checkups.

A healthy lifestyle has several other benefits: it will make you feel younger, stronger, and more energetic.

In fact, a recent publication noted that after the age of fifty-five, the chance of getting a stroke doubles every ten years!

can cause paralysis and death. Diabetes also can accelerate the atherosclerosis process.

These reasons alone make diabetes a risk factor for stroke, but there's more:

- A person with diabetes is up to three times more likely to have a stroke.

- Studies have found that people with diabetes are twice as likely to have hypertension than those without the disease.

- Another study found that 42 percent of people who had strokes also had diabetes.

- The combination of hypertension and diabetes is much more common among African-Americans and Hispanics.

- Diabetics are also more prone to obesity and high cholesterol levels.

Like aging, there is little we can do to prevent inherited diabetes. But we can control it through medication, diet, exercise, and a healthy lifestyle.

Cholesterol Levels

We all talk about it. We check labels for it. We get our blood checked for it. But many of us are not quite sure what cholesterol is—or its connection to disease.

Basically, cholesterol is a waxy material that the body manufactures, and, believe it or not, it's natural and necessary for many of our functions. But today, there can be too much of a good thing. Not only does the body manufacture cholesterol, but cholesterol also is found in many of the foods we eat, such as steak and eggs. And saturated fats found in such foods as meat, cheese, milk fat, shortening, and even margarine contribute even more to higher blood cholesterol levels than does dietary intake of cholesterol.

And excess spells trouble. Here's why.

Cholesterol is carried in the bloodstream by lipoproteins, a "shopping cart" substance of fat and protein produced by the liver. The lipoprotein that does most of the work is low-density lipoprotein (LDL) cholesterol. All well and good, but once the body has taken what it needs, the LDL is still floating around, all dressed up with nowhere to go. Eventually, this floating LDL cholesterol settles on the artery walls, clogging passageways or causing clots that could break off and travel to the brain. This is why LDL is called "bad cholesterol."

But LDL does not travel alone. There is a "good cholesterol" at work as well: high-density lipoprotein (HDL). HDL carries cholesterol back to the liver for processing and elimination. Like

A Vital Connection

Studies have found that for every 6-millimeter mercury decrease in diastolic blood pressure, there is a 40-percent reduction in the incidence of stroke. One way to help to reduce your risk of stroke? Losing weight.

a minute Dustbuster, HDL suctions up the cholesterol left by the LDL and helps clear the arteries.

The risk of high cholesterol comes from the amount of LDL in the bloodstream. Cholesterol has received most of its press from its relationship with heart attacks. Indeed, until recently, cholesterol has not been considered a risk for stroke. But new research has shown that lowering cholesterol is important in stroke prevention. A recent study of the new "statin" drugs showed that by lowering LDL cholesterol by 23 percent to 42 percent, the risk of stroke was decreased by 29 percent.

In short, cholesterol levels, especially LDL cholesterol, must be watched. The current recommendation is keep your cholesterol below 200MG/DL, and if your LDL is more than 100MG/DL you should be on a statin medication. High-risk patients with multiple risk factors should try to get their LDL down to 70MG/DL. And if your levels are high, help decrease the numbers by eating a low-fat diet, taking cholesterol-lowering medication, and exercising regularly. You are never too young to know your cholesterol level and to start working on a healthy lifestyle.

Heart Disease History

It makes sense. If there are problems in the heart, there is the potential for problems in the brain. Remember, blood clots can form in the heart, then travel to the brain—closing off the arteries and causing a stroke.

Usually our hearts beat in a monotonous but reassuring regular rhythm. But, particularly as we age, they may adopt a highly irregular beat called **atrial fibrillation.** These irregular beats of the atrium are less efficient, and blood clots can form in the heart, poised and ready to head to the brain. A person with atrial fibrillation is 4 percent to 18 percent more likely to have a stroke. The

Chapter 2   *Risk Factors*   39

good news is that blood "thinners" like Coumadin® (see Chapter 10 for a complete description) can significantly reduce the risk of stroke.

In some cases, blood clots may form on a damaged heart valve. Diseases like rheumatic fever can leave roughened, floppy heart valves that attract small bits of debris and blood clots. At other times, a heart attack may leave a section of the heart muscle weakened—another magnet for those dangerous blood clots that might break off and travel to the brain.

The Ills of Tobacco Smoking

Smoking

- damages the walls of the arteries over the long term

- narrows the small blood passageways in the brain

- reduces the amount of nourishing oxygen in the blood

- affects circulation

It is a fact—smoking doubles the risk of having a stroke. That's right, you are twice as likely to have a disabling stroke if you smoke. Smoking has a major distinction: it is the most preventable of all the risks for stroke.

Simple. But, as anyone who has ever smoked knows, quitting is easier said than done. Even though studies have found that smokers are one and one-half to three times more at risk for stroke than nonsmokers, even though smoking adversely affects circulation and blood supply, and even though the risk of smoking is high with or without taking into account high blood pressure, heart disease, and age, many people continue to smoke.

It has been estimated that 61,000 strokes could be prevented each year if cigarette smoking was eliminated.

Thousands of people have quit, and even if you are not successful the first or second time, try, try again. Contact the American Lung Association, the American Cancer Society, or your local hospital for smoking-cessation programs, suggestions, and support.

If you smoke, you must quit. It can save your life.

Taking Birth Control Pills

Birth control pills have helped shape the way we think, the way we act, and, obviously, the way we conceive. They helped give birth to women's rights. They influenced an entire generation of young adults.

But as the years pass, studies have found that there are some side effects with oral contraceptives.

One of these is the risk of stroke, especially in women over the age of thirty who have a history of hypertension and smoking. One study of stroke in young women discovered that certain women who used birth control pills were at an increased risk for stroke compared to women who did not. This risk increased in women who have hypertension. And other studies show there is also a connection between oral contraceptives, heavy cigarette smoking, and stroke. The overall risk is quite small, so you need to weigh it against the fact that pregnancy itself carries a risk. The decision is difficult, but women who are older, hypertensive, and smoke should consult their doctors regarding the risks of taking birth control pills.

We've reached the end of our risk factor list. As you can see, some of these risks are preventable—and others are not. But studies have shown without a doubt that the prevalence of stroke has dropped in recent years because hypertension is being success-fully treated with medication.

Unfortunately, this decline has plateaued recently, which further shows that other risk factors must be treated as well. A lower-fat diet that is also lower in salt, exercise, weight loss, no smoking, even taking one drink of alcohol a day (but don't forget that heavy drinking increases the risk of stroke!)—all these can help reduce the risk of stroke.

And reducing one risk factor can have a favorable outcome on the others. As we have seen, many conditions are related: high cholesterol and hypertension, obesity and diabetes. Treating one of these factors can help treat another.

An ounce of prevention is worth many pounds of cure.

You now know the "why" of stroke. Now it's time to discover the "how," with facts and insights into the three basic types of stroke.

CHAPTER 3

The Types of Strokes

"It happened so quickly, like a bolt out of the blue."

—*Wife of a seventy-year-old retired salesman who had a stroke*

Ginger, an only child, was very close to her father. It had been only the two of them for years now, ever since her mother died of cancer.

Now, it wasn't as if she saw him all the time. Although they lived within fifteen minutes of each other, both led very active lives. Ginger worked and lived in Manhattan. Her father was a prominent ophthalmologist in Connecticut. Although he already was in his late sixties, he had no desire to retire. He loved his work; he was good at it.

Occasionally, Ginger would accompany her father to various functions. Even though he dated many women, he never wanted to settle down. He had loved his wife. Period. And he loved Ginger.

To see each other more, Ginger and her dad made plans to meet once a month, on a Sunday. They would sometimes go shopping. They would go for a walk along the river. They played golf. And sometimes, they merely enjoyed brunch at a country restaurant.

This particular Sunday, Ginger was to meet her dad at Grey's Country Inn, a favorite restaurant of theirs. She arrived a few minutes early, so she wasn't overly concerned that her father hadn't arrived yet.

Ginger ordered a Bloody Mary and sat by the stone fireplace; she chatted with the owner. But by the time she had finished her drink, her dad was fifteen minutes late. As a doctor, he'd always been punctual. She started to get concerned.

Her anxiety grew as fifteen minutes turned into forty-five minutes. She called the house several times, only to get her father's answering machine. She called his service; he'd left no message for her, nor had he had any emergencies.

Her heart heavy with fear and anticipation, Ginger got into her car. She drove to his house, a good half hour away. Her dad's Toyota was in the garage. The Sunday newspaper was still on the lawn.

Ginger opened the front door with her key. "Dad!" she screamed, ready to yell at him for giving her such a scare. Silence. She ran up the stairs and into his bedroom. "Dad . . . "

The bed was empty; it was unmade. She started to run into his bathroom but stopped short. There, on the carpet between the bed and the bathroom, was her father, face down, still in his pajamas, sprawled on the carpet.

Ginger's father had died of a stroke, a bolt out of the blue that left his daughter in shock.

For Ginger, the type of stroke her father suffered meant nothing. But for doctors, scientists, and rehabilitation-treatment teams, the type of stroke is vital for proper diagnosis and outcome prognosis. For a loved one who survives a stroke, impaired but thankfully alive, the type of stroke, along with its location and severity, can make all the difference between a poor outcome and a successful rehabilitation plan.

The Supreme Drought: Infarction

No, this isn't some sci-fi movie title. An infarction is a deadly condition that occurs in stroke.

It is, quite simply, a condition in which the brain cells die.

Here's how infarction occurs:

1. An artery becomes clogged in either the brain or the neck.

2. Blood, with its life-sustaining oxygen, cannot get past the clogged-up passageway.

3. The brain cells beyond that clog literally die from lack of blood and oxygen.

4. The function those dead cells controlled is now gone.

Because of the configuration of arteries in the brain, the area hit by the "drought" usually forms a wedge shape. Visualize it as the sprinkler system you use on your lawn. If one sprinkler head malfunctions, the wedge of grass it watered will die.

As with all other aspects of stroke, location is everything. Small or large might not be important with infarction. Rather, it is where the infarction took place that decides a person's fate. Even a small infarction can cause severe disability if it occurs in a vital area. If the brain tissue dies in the interior area of the brain, it can cause paralysis on one-half of the body. If it is in the occipital lobe area, it can affect vision.

But the subsequent infarction is only part of the story. There is also its beginning—and the two types of stroke that can create the "drought."

Thrombotic Beat

It's called a **thrombosis,** the most common form of stroke. In fact, 80–85 percent of all strokes are ischemic in nature. Here, the blood flow in the brain, either deep in its interior or in the less deep carotid artery in the neck, is blocked because of a clot that forms in the artery. Atherosclerosis is its greatest influence. Think of it. Either through cholesterol deposits or aging, the inside walls of the arteries become less flexible; thick deposits of fat form, and passageways become too narrow for blood to flow through smoothly. Instead, the blood forms a clot around these thick deposits as it tries to get past.

Ironically, these clots usually begin as a healthy measure. The deposits or rough places on the artery wall are seen by the body as a "call to arms," a need to stave off infection. The blood, thinking these areas need repair, clots around them. Platelets send out their thin clotting fibers. Red and white blood cells join in the action. Soon, the clotting has a life of its own, acting like a net as it pulls platelets, red blood cells, even bits of floating cholesterol into its web. A scab can form, making the mass of cholesterol and blood even thicker.

The result? A clogged-up passageway that life-sustaining blood can't pass through.

The ultimate result? A thrombotic stroke.

Embolic Action

This type of stroke, too, is caused by a clot. These embolic strokes are less common than their thrombotic cousin. But these clots, called emboli, are the traveling salespeople of stroke, a mass of tissue, blood, and cholesterol that originates somewhere else in our body, usually in the heart or the neck's carotid artery, only to end up in the brain. Here, when the clotting action occurs, a piece of clot eventually breaks off. This clot, or **embolism,** is carried by the bloodstream to the brain, where the arteries are smaller. Soon, the clot gets stuck, literally plugging up the passageway beyond it. Blood simply cannot get past the embolism.

A third type of stroke has less to do with infarction's "drought" than it has to do with flooding.

A Hemorrhaging Landscape

Only 10 percent of all strokes are hemorrhagic. But hemorrhagic strokes are also the most deadly. There is good news, however: studies have found that if people survive hemorrhagic strokes, they can make the greatest and most dramatic gains over time in rehabilitation.

Hemorrhagic strokes usually are helped along by hypertension, which weakens and changes the artery walls in the brain. A weakened wall eventually ruptures, spilling blood into the brain. Sometimes this problem is congenital, a condition that has existed since birth. Unfortunately, high blood pressure can stretch this already vulnerable wall to its limits. In the same way a worn tire can explode one day while you are driving, this wall can ultimately burst. We call this medical "blowout" a ruptured **aneurysm**—which sends blood all around the surface of the brain.

Blood Flood

There are two types of hemorrhagic strokes. One is called subarachnoid hemorrhage, or SAH, which occurs in the area surrounding the brain. This occurs when aneurysms or arteriovenous (artery and vein) malformations rupture. There may be no warning, except an acute and extremely severe headache.

The other type of hemorrhage is called intracerebral hemorrhage, or ICH. This stroke usually occurs deep within the regions of the brain, and its symptoms vary, depending on the function it has affected. ICH strokes are caused most often by hypertension.

Little Lacunes

Think of lacunar strokes as tiny infarctions. Smaller than one cubic centimeter in size, they occur where the larger arteries branch off into the minute vessels, or capillaries, deep within the brain.

But like all strokes, location is everything. Lacunes can pack a big wallop if they occur in critical areas. Only one tiny lacune, deep inside the brain, can lead to total paralysis on one side. On the other hand, lacunes can go unnoticed until their numbers increase and more and more brain tissue is lost.

Lacunar strokes are most common in patients who have diabetes or hypertension. This type of stroke accounts for approximately 25 percent of all strokes.

These are the different types of strokes. Their signs and symptoms vary, based on location, type, and severity.

Once a stroke occurs, we deal with the consequences. But most important of all is recognizing the indicator called a transient ischemic attack (TIA)—and seeking medical attention to possibly stop a full-blown stroke from happening.

CHAPTER 4

Warning Signs

"I had this numbness and it didn't feel right.
Honest to God, if I hadn't contacted my
doctor, I might have had a stroke."
— *A healthy fifty-two-year-old accountant*

A stroke doesn't always just come out of nowhere. Warning signs can be recognized and treated before a full-fledged stroke occurs—if you know how to read them.

Fact: only 15 percent of stroke patients have a history of transient ischemic attacks (TIAs).

Fact: the symptoms of TIAs are frequently ignored by the patient.

Fact: these symptoms usually develop rapidly and frequently disappear within fifteen minutes.

Fact: If an MRI scan is performed, it will show that one third of TIA patients actually have had a stroke.

Fact: 20 percent of people who have TIAs will have a full-fledged stroke within ten years, unless their symptoms are treated.

Fact: only a small percentage of the population is educated enough about strokes to recognize a stroke when it occurs.

All these facts point to one bottom line: if recognized and treated, TIAs can prevent a full-fledged stroke from taking place. But note the crucial phrase: "if recognized and treated." Unfortunately, diagnosing a TIA is easier said than done. Although getting immediate help and seeking immediate medical attention is paramount, most people who suffer a stroke do not seek help until they've had their symptoms for more than eight hours.

It's up to you to make that first step, to understand when your body is in danger, and to reach out for medical care.

To that end, here's a brief lesson in transient ischemic attacks, the powerful warnings that, if heeded, might stop tragedy before it begins.

TIAs

Although the phrase *transient ischemic attacks* sounds complicated, its meaning is fairly straightforward. A TIA is a temporary interruption in the blood supply to a portion of the brain, which usually doesn't last more than a few minutes or a few hours.

TIAs can be caused by traveling clots, just as in full-fledged strokes, or they can be caused by clogged-up artery walls. In fact, the only difference between a TIA and a stroke is that a TIA is

Symptoms of TIA and Stroke: The Short List

- Sudden numbness or weakness of the face, arm or leg, especially on one side of the body
- Sudden confusion, trouble speaking or understanding
- Sudden trouble walking, dizziness, loss of balance or coordination
- Sudden trouble seeing in one or both eyes
- Sudden severe headache with no known cause

temporary. Clots or clogging deposits eventually are broken up or dissolved.

But before the clot or deposit disappears, symptoms may appear. As with a completed stroke, the symptoms of TIA also depend on the area of the brain where the blood supply was interrupted. Unfortunately, because these symptoms disappear, sometimes within minutes, they are often ignored. Furthermore, because they are often vague or mild, we quickly ignore them. After all, who wants to believe that they could be having a stroke?

But therein lies the danger of TIA. Yes, its symptoms fade, *but the underlying mechanisms that created it still are hidden within our bodies.* Blood still can be filled with cholesterol. Artery walls still can be vulnerable. Clots still can be forming.

For a TIA to be an effective warning, *medical intervention is crucial.* This is an emergency.

Period.

Preventive measures for hypertension, diabetes, or any of the controllable risk factors that we've talked about in earlier chapters can be initiated only if a physician is made aware of your TIA symptoms—as inconsequential as you yourself might find them.

To help in your personal TIA awareness quest, here are the most common symptoms:

In the Eye of the Beholder

Only you can bring your symptoms to the attention of a physician. But she also must ask the right questions to help discover those symptoms that point to TIA—and those that indicate something else. Good diagnostic skills are crucial. It's not so important to know that your hand was numb as it is to know how long the numbness lasted. It's not as key to simply know that you felt dizzy as it is to know under what circumstances you experienced such discomfort. Your doctor will know how to diagnose properly; she will know what questions to ask.

Temporary weakness, numbness, or paralysis of the hand, arm, leg, or face on one or both sides of the body. These are the most crucial "red flag" symptoms. They are not only the most common characteristics of TIA, but if immediately brought to your physician's attention, they can save your life. One note: this weakness or numbness is not the same thing as the "pins and needles" you feel when, for example, your foot falls asleep. It comes on quickly and leaves just as fast.

Sudden blurred, dimmed, or complete loss of vision in one or both eyes that lasts longer than a few seconds. Sudden loss of vision in one eye can signal an embolus to the main artery to the eye, and the loss of vision in both eyes can be the result of inadequate blood flow to the occipital lobes.

Speech and language difficulties. This can involve having trouble actually speaking and understanding the spoken word (aphasia) or the written word (alexia). Slurred or "thick" speech (dysarthria) is a sign of a vertebrobasilar TIA, which is a TIA in the arteries at the back of the brain.

Lack of coordination or balance. Technically, this condition is yet another *A* term: **ataxia.** It can involve arms or legs—resulting in difficulty holding a glass or walking. It is a sign of vertebrobasilar insufficiency.

Hollenhorst's Contribution

His name might not mean anything to you, but Robert W. Hollenhorst was the first doctor to see cholesterol in the back of the eye. By looking at the eye, a doctor can detect the presence of a bright yellow crystal (which traveled from either the carotid artery in the neck or from the heart) within a small artery. This is an indicator for a stroke and requires immediate attention.

Vertigo. Dizziness is one of the most common symptoms of vertebrobasilar TIA, affecting the back of the brain where the vertebral and basal arteries reside. Seventy percent of all people who have this type of TIA experience this dizziness. But vertigo must be combined with other symptoms for it to signify an attack. For example, dizziness without numbness, weakness, or speech problems is rarely a sign of TIA.

Nausea or vomiting or both. Alone, these symptoms are too vague to point to TIA, but in combination with vertigo, speech problems, or loss of balance, they can signal a possible attack.

A transient ischemic attack is reversible. Heeding its warning signs can go far in preventing a stroke. But sometimes the "dreaded impossible" occurs, despite our best intentions and our best care.

Sometimes a stroke will strike—and in the next section, we'll see exactly what symptoms it creates and, most important, how it can be treated.

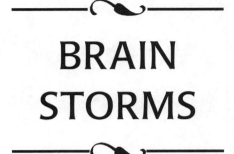

PART II

BRAIN STORMS

CHAPTER 5

When Stroke Strikes

"The worst part was the feeling that I was alone. I knew that people have strokes every day, but that didn't really comfort me. I couldn't help it. I felt like mine was different, that nobody really understood."

—*A seventy-four-year-old stroke patient*

Some of the most devastating elements of stroke occur in its aftermath—the silence, the paralysis, the inability to perform ordinary routines. These are some of the profound aftershocks of stroke:

- When Joan's speech therapist asked her if she wanted to leave the rehabilitation hospital soon, Joan replied: "Beggin bog I no lali someday lud." Amid the gibberish, Joan's therapist could discern actual words—and hope. But it still would take time for Joan to recover her ability to communicate.

- Morris wanted to move his left arm. He was determined to move his left arm. And, indeed, if sheer will were enough, he would have moved his arm a hundred times. But despite his desire, despite the requests from his occupational therapist, he couldn't do it. His left arm was a heavy, paralyzed weight.

- Cynthia was weary of her feeding tube. Inside, in her mind, she was sitting around a dining room table with those she loved. She was eating and drinking and laughing. She was in a place where swallowing was as natural to her as breathing, as blinking her eyes. But Cynthia's recent stroke changed all that. She literally had to retrain her body to function.

- Johnson knew he was depressed. He knew all the signs—the hopelessness, the weariness, the lack of appetite, the loss of sleep. But none of these symptoms mattered. In fact, nothing mattered. Johnson, like 30 percent to 50 percent of all people who have a stroke, was suffering from a poststroke depression. And unless it was treated, his depression would affect his rehabilitation. It would interfere with his motivation and his progress.

As highly individual as all of us are, as different and unique as our separate memories, perceptions, and feelings are, when stroke strikes, many of its symptoms are universal. Paralysis, depression, an inability to communicate—as the previously mentioned examples show, there is a commonality among stroke damage.

And this damage depends on locale. It's not just a matter of when stroke occurs or how it happens. Actual symptoms are a function of *where* stroke strikes.

How We Speak

Speech often is affected when a stroke strikes, and the resulting speech disturbance often depends on the distribution of communication skills between the left and the right hemispheres of the brain.

As a rule of thumb, if you are right-handed, most of your language skills are located in the left side of your brain. If you are left-handed, there is a 50-percent chance that your language abilities will be in your right hemisphere.

Stroke Location

As we have seen, the type of stroke a person has is a crucial element in its degree of severity and in its symptoms.

The location of the stroke is the other crucial element.

It's a fact: most strokes occur in only one side, or hemisphere, of the brain. And their symptoms will appear on only one side of the body, the side *opposite* the affected hemisphere in the brain. In other words, when a stroke strikes the right hemisphere of the brain, it will affect the left side of the body. When a stroke strikes the left hemisphere of the brain, it will affect the body's right side.

The Number-One Symptom

The most common symptom of stroke is paralysis on one side of the body. This phenomenon can be total or partial, affecting, for example, the fine motor movements of our hands and feet or creating a numbness or paralysis in our entire leg or arm. Further, it is not unusual to have total paralysis of a hand or foot but still be able to move a shoulder or hip.

Other Symptoms

Numbness or paralysis, however, is only one part of the story. Each hemisphere also controls different thinking, speaking, and information-processing functions. A stroke in the right hemisphere can affect, for example, memory, attention span, and impulse control. A stroke in the left side of the brain can affect language skills and cognition, which is, literally, the act of knowing.

But not every stroke is found in the right or left hemisphere of the brain. As with most situations, there are exceptions to every rule. Although less common than their "right-left" counterparts, some strokes occur in the brain stem or in the cerebellum. Strokes here may affect movement, balance, and basic body functions, such as swallowing and breathing.

Of course, we usually don't see every symptom in every person who suffers a stroke. Nor are every person's symptoms the same. But when stroke strikes a specific area, there are enough similarities to make pinpointing the location a help in diagnosis and, ultimately, in the rehabilitation outcome. Thus, in the next few chapters, we will discuss briefly the common symptoms that are found in right-hemisphere, left-hemisphere, and brain stem and cerebellar strokes.

CHAPTER 6

Right-Hemisphere Stroke

> "It was the little things. They didn't happen
> all the time, but when they did, it was hard.
> Like crying suddenly or talking nonstop.
> Or suddenly not recognizing me, even if it
> just lasted for a moment. Yes, that was the
> hardest. Not seeing me."
>
> *—Husband of a sixty-two-year-old stroke patient*

When Ed woke up, he was in a hospital room. An oxygen mask lay on his face. Fluid was dripping into his arm. He was disoriented; he began to thrash his head. He tried to move his left arm. He couldn't. A nurse came over to him.

He wanted to say, "Help me!" but he didn't have the strength. The nurse tried to calm him; he fell back to sleep. Later, Ed would remember the backyard right before it happened. It had been a bright Sunday afternoon. A soft breeze had blown through the maple trees; soft jazz had been playing on the radio, filtering through from the kitchen. He'd been barbecuing some hamburgers on the grill when the headache began. He dropped the spatula. He fell down, unconscious, on the grass.

Ed had suffered a stroke. After performing a series of diagnostic tests in the hospital, his physicians were able to be more specific: Ed had suffered a stroke because of a thrombus in his right middle cerebral artery. Damage had been done in his right temporal and frontal lobes and deep in the thalamic region of his brain as well.

Ed was a victim of a right-hemisphere stroke, with its own set of symptoms, its own characteristics, that, in time, would either improve or become a part of his life.

Right-Brain Characteristics

As we have seen, the right and left hemispheres of the brain control different functions. But like most things in life, they aren't divided neatly in two. They work in concert, one adding dimension to the other, one overlapping the other within every aspect of our personality—from thinking to speaking, from performing to perceiving.

But depending on the specific function, one side does dominate the other.

The right hemisphere is more in control of our visual organization, perception, and attention. It adds meaning and substance to what we see.

The right brain also is responsible for nonverbal communication, for the slang, inflection, style, and gestures that go along with our conversations with others.

Furthermore, our right hemisphere also is involved in our ability to perceive space, to understand where we are, what we are looking at, what we are doing, and why various objects are placed where they are.

All these functions are affected when a stroke occurs in the right hemisphere of the brain. Using Ed as our prototype, let's now go over these "right blights," these most common right-hemisphere stroke symptoms.

Right-Brain Stroke Symptom One: Paralysis or Weakness on the Left, or Opposite, Side of the Body

When Ed's family first heard the word **hemiparesis,** they didn't understand what it meant. They soon learned that it meant weakness, and that along with **hemiplegia,** or paralysis, it was the most common symptom of stroke.

Because Ed's stroke occurred in his right hemisphere, his weakness was seen on his left side. He could not move his left hand well; he found it difficult to hold a utensil or tie a shoe. He also found walking a chore at first.

Gradually, through rehabilitation, Ed grew stronger. But at the same time, his muscles became spastic. As one muscle group in his left arm became more toned and stronger, another remained weak. This imbalance caused his hand to clench into a tight fist and his left arm to flex tightly against his chest. His leg would even draw up on him at night as he lay in bed. Fortunately, his spasticity improved with medication and splints.

Right-Brain Stroke Symptom Two: Perception Problems, Both Visual and Spatial

Getting dressed was a chore for Ed—and not only because of his weakened state. He knew something wasn't right with his shirt, but he couldn't connect it with the fact that it was inside out. He couldn't understand how to use the buttons or where to put his socks. This is called **dressing apraxia,** a defect in visuomotor orientation resulting from right parietal lobe damage.

Besides dressing, there is showering, eating meals, shopping, brushing your teeth—all these activities of daily living that we take for granted can become monumental challenges for people

A List of Right-Hemisphere Stroke Symptoms

- Numbness or weakness on the left side of the body
- Difficulty in performing daily tasks
- Perception difficulties
- Neglect of left side
- Visual memory impairment
- Excessive talking
- Short attention span
- Poor judgment
- Time disorientation
- Loss of left visual field
- Impaired abstract thinking
- Extreme emotional highs and lows
- Lethargy
- Impulsiveness

who suffer a stroke. And because the right brain governs our ability to recognize visual and spatial cues, it makes sense that we would have difficulty with tasks that require us to see the relationship of one thing to another.

Thus, Ed, and others like him, will have difficulty recognizing the route to the restroom, the order in which to eat a meal, or the symbols on a map. He also will have trouble copying or sketching something; he won't be able to place it in its proper form on a piece of paper.

And to add to the confusion, Ed also temporarily lost his left visual field (**hemianopsia**). Because he couldn't see his shirt crumpled on a chair in the left-hand corner of his room without turning his head, Ed assumed it was missing.

Right-Brain Stroke Symptom Three: Neglect and Denial

Neglect can mean many things. It can mean a failure to focus on the outside world. Or a lack of attention. Or, in its extreme, an inability to recognize that one has even had a stroke.

In 1981, Dr. M. Mesulam isolated the attention network in the brain. He found that the small reticular formation, found deep within the brain stem, is responsible for general arousal and wakefulness. The parietal lobes concern themselves with sensory cues, and the frontal lobes help coordinate our actual activities. The limbic system provides the necessary desire and motivation to interact with our environment.

Disruption in any of these brain areas will cause problems in attention that can cause neglect. And because the right hemisphere contains the neurons that get the entire attention network going, it makes sense that a right-sided stroke will stop attention in its tracks.

Thus, although they might have appeared bizarre, Ed's reactions were typical. He would shave only the right side of his face. He ate only the food on the right side of his dinner plate. He didn't notice anyone who approached him from the left. We have seen other patients draw only half a figure when asked to copy a

From the Greek

Neglect caused by right-hemisphere stroke can take on an extreme form. When a patient denies his symptoms or the stroke itself, this is called **anosognosia.** You can show the person their paralyzed arm and ask them who it belongs to and they will not realize that it is their own arm!

On a larger scale of "denial of illness," the person doesn't believe or recognize that there is anything wrong with him. This makes rehabilitation very difficult.

A Neglect Test

It's important to realize that the neglect of the left side is *independent* of any other symptoms of right-hemisphere stroke. It may or may not have anything to do with any other visual, processing, or sensory deficits. But recognizing neglect—and knowing whether it stands alone or in concert with other symptoms—is crucial for successful rehabilitation.

How does a rehabilitation therapist discover what is neglect and what is not? Here are some simple tests:

- A patient is asked to draw a clock face, including the numerical hours, or a daisy with petals. A person suffering from neglect might completely omit the left side of his flower or clock.

- A patient is asked to circle every letter *A* that she can find on a piece of paper. If her symptoms include neglect, she may ignore each *A* on the left side of the paper.

- The therapist stands behind the patient and snaps his fingers, first on the left side, then on the right side, and then on both sides at the same time. This way he can determine if neglect includes auditory stimuli.

- When the therapist moves her fingers within, first, the patient's left visual field, and then within the patient's right, the therapist can determine if neglect is combined with any visual field deficits.

picture. We have seen still others neglect the left syllable in different words, seeing and saying "ball" instead of "baseball," "loon" instead of "balloon."

Neglect is a major issue in right-hemisphere strokes, and it is a difficult one for families to understand. Denying the left side of the body, refusing to believe that his arm is paralyzed or that it even belongs to him, can severely slow progress. After all, if you don't recognize the fact that you have a problem, it will be difficult to work on it.

But there is good news. We have seen patients "blossom" months later, their neglect completely and spontaneously clearing.

Right-Brain Stroke Symptom Four: Visual Memory Problems

When a stroke hits the thalamus or the right temporal lobe, visual memory can be affected. What does this mean? For Ed, it meant that when he tried to read the newspaper in the morning with his coffee, he would forget what he'd read by his second sip. It also meant that he forgot what his bedroom looked like, what picture hung in the front hall, and, for the first few weeks of his recuperation, what he looked like in the mirror. This extreme inability to recognize your own face or the face of someone you love is called **prosopagnosia** and is manifested by patients who have had strokes in the occipital and temporal regions of both brain halves. They will recognize people only by the sound of their voices.

Right-Brain Stroke Symptom Five: Aphasia, or Language Deficits

Although the left hemisphere controls most of our basic language skills, from vocabulary to pronunciation, the right hemisphere provides its color. Indeed, studies have shown that to rebuild language skills, rehabilitation teams must include nonverbal, right-brain–oriented programs. Patients who have suffered a right-brain stroke might lose their speech inflection; their words might come out flat. Similarly, they might not be able to pick up the inflection, emotion, or meaning of someone else's conversation. In scientific terms, **prosody** is the color that we add to our statements that make them questions or exclamations. **Aprosody** is its loss, a result of right-brain stroke.

Ed had something a little different but no less uncommon in his right-hemisphere stroke. He lost the ability to use his hands and face, to gesture, while he spoke. But there was some good news. He still could understand the gestures of others.

There's one more symptom that deals with language, one that can, understandably, try a loved one's nerves: excessive talking. Ed chattered nonstop during meals. As soon as someone else stopped talking, he began.

Right-Brain Stroke Symptom Six: Poor Judgment

It makes sense. Sensory impairment, memory loss, neglect, lack of attention—these separate symptoms of stroke can, unfortunately, culminate in other symptoms, such as time disorientation, impaired abstract thinking, and, ultimately, poor judgment. This inability to judge and decipher events and situations is particularly dangerous because, more times than not, it shows itself when it comes to safety measures.

Walking out of the house in a bathrobe and slippers; getting behind the wheel of a car without a license, glasses, or a sense of direction; preparing lunch in the kitchen without recognizing the difference between dishwasher powder and salt—all these are hazardous to a stroke patient's health.

Before Ed was able to leave the hospital, his family had to be counseled regarding his physical safety needs. His home had to be made safe. And they had to arrange for someone to be with Ed twenty-four hours a day.

Right-Brain Stroke Symptom Seven: Emotional Problems

Ed's family couldn't keep up. He'd go from laughter to tears in seconds. Extreme emotional highs and lows are common in right-hemisphere strokes, but mood imbalance can be eased through medication, patience, understanding—and time.

These, then, in brief, are the symptoms of right-hemisphere stroke. But right is right and left is left. There is a difference. Let's go on to the symptoms of left-hemisphere stroke now.

CHAPTER 7

Left-Hemisphere Stroke

"I don't know what was worse. The stroke
itself or the fact that I just didn't care what
happened. I was so depressed."

—*A seventy-nine-year-old veterinarian
who had a left-hemisphere stroke*

Mary was sorting her mail at her desk when her right hand felt numb. It wasn't bad, similar to other times the last few days. She rubbed her hand and gave it no notice.

But Mary's mind soon began to wander; she felt light and unfocused. She looked out her office window. She noticed the men and women in the windows across the way, the men without jackets, their ties flying as they walked from office to office. She could almost hear the women's high heels clicking on the floor. They look liked miniature, mechanical figures, like a music box. "Like a music box," Mary thought, before she lost her breath, before the headache blinded her, before she fell unconscious, scattering her just-sorted mail on her polished desk.

Mary had just experienced what physicians call a cerebral infarction, or a completed stroke. According to her doctor, she had had a series of TIAs as well, a series of warning signs, including numbness, light-headedness, and speech problems that she had, unfortunately, ignored.

At sixty-five, Mary was a strong, robust woman; she had been a private financial counselor for an international banking concern. She spoke five languages; she handled mathematical projections easily and was a master of numbers.

Luckily, Mary survived her stroke. But her luck fell short when it came to location. Her stroke was concentrated in the middle cerebral artery of the left hemisphere, which meant that her executive functions, her ability to organize, focus, and plan ahead, were disabled. So was her proficiency in math and language.

Left-Brain Characteristics

All was not bleak, however. There was good news for Mary. Her rehabilitation team was confident that her brain would improve, that many of the injured neurons would become active once more, that the network of neurons in the brain might find another route to implement the same function. Combined with the retraining program in the hospital, Mary's physicians felt that she would, in time, lead a full, if different, life again.

This was no cockeyed optimism at work. The rehabilitation team was experienced and well trained in stroke treatment. They were no strangers to left-hemisphere stroke, and they had successfully treated patients such as Mary over and over again. Indeed, the symptoms Mary displayed are common when stroke hits the left brain.

As we have seen in Chapter 1, the left hemisphere controls our language skills, our verbal communications, our use of logic and rational thought.

It's also true, as we have seen, that the left hemisphere works in concert with the right, and that language and comprehension skills are found in both. But, here, in the left hemisphere, speech disturbances come out in different ways: words might not be understood nor physically produced.

Depression, too, is more common in left-hemisphere stroke than when stroke strikes the supposedly more emotional right side. Using Mary as our prototype, let's go over these and the other symptoms unique to left-hemisphere injury, the "left behinds" of stroke.

Left-Brain Stroke Symptom One: Paralysis or Weakness on the Right Side of the Body

One of the first things Mary noticed when she regained consciousness was that she could not move her right arm. It felt like dead weight, an alien object. Furthermore, her right leg was very weak. She could move it up slightly, an inch or two from her bed, but only with a great deal of energy. The right side of her face was paralyzed.

As we have seen in right-hemisphere stroke, paralysis or weakness on the opposite side of the body is a common symptom and one that can improve with time and proper rehabilitation. Within four weeks, Mary could move her right leg up off the bed. She could begin to move the fingers on her right hand. She even walked in the parallel bars during physical therapy.

Although Mary did not have this problem, other patients may experience the loss of their right-side visual field. Like their right-hemisphere stroke counterparts, they cannot see anything on their opposite side.

Still other patients can become confused between right and left, even though they do not have a visual field loss. Right shoes are put on left feet; therapy can be confusing not knowing which side is which.

Left-Brain Stroke Symptom Two: Language Difficulties

As with right-hemisphere stroke, language disabilities are bound to crop up in left-sided strokes. But rather than attacking color and inflection, the problem will be much more grounded in actual speech itself.

Mary could not express herself. When she wanted a glass of water, she found herself saying, "Cou I diz say stove?" Sometimes she couldn't articulate single words at all. She found herself pointing to the glass instead of speaking. Within a few days, Mary was able to communicate to her speech therapist by a combination of two- and three-word phrases and hand gestures. But it would take time until Mary could form sentences again—and more time until she could read or write clearly.

A List of Left-Hemisphere Stroke Symptoms

- Numbness or weakness on the right side of the body
- Partial or complete loss of speaking or understanding language
- Impaired thought processing, including decreased problem-solving ability, poor judgment, and an inability to see errors
- Confusion between left and right
- Lack of insight
- Loss of the visual field on the right
- Decreased memory
- Slowness
- Depression

Left-hemisphere language difficulties, or **aphasia,** can take other forms. In fact, approximately 85,000 of those Americans who are stricken by stroke every year suffer aphasia. Mary had a nonfluent aphasia with an ability to say only a few words. Other people might have a fluent aphasia where they have many words available and they can also make up phrases. One of our patients would say "spoof " instead of "spoon" and "prazum" instead of "please."

Others might experience the following:

Repeat phrases over and over again. A former stroke patient of ours would, at one time, declare, "Hallo, hallo, hallo," at any time and at any place, despite the situation. When a nurse would come in to change his linen, he'd say, "Hallo, hallo, hallo." When a visitor would get up from a chair to leave, he'd say, "Hallo, hallo, hallo." When he first went home, he found himself repeating this phrase over and over again—in the supermarket, on the street, and over dinner.

Hear something other than what you said. Another patient of ours could pronounce his words just fine. But he couldn't understand much of what we said. To him, our conversations were gobbledygook, a foreign language that he couldn't penetrate. Instead of "Good morning, Mr. Smith. How are you today?" he heard something else—the gist of which we may never know.

Suffer from Broca's (nonfluent) aphasia. These patients will, like Mary, have problems speaking. Their conversations will be slow, full of effort, and ungrammatical. Initially, they will not be able to write or be able to read more than a few words.

Have trouble picking out individual words. One of our patients, a middle-aged woman, could speak just fine. She could understand what others said to her. But put a book, a magazine, or a newspaper in front of her and, without directions, she was at a loss. She would read a sentence or two and then blank out on

Tying the Knot: An Observation

The observation below comes from a man, a stroke patient, who, for forty years, had donned a bow tie every day. Two months after his stroke, he tried it again. It took him ten tries to tie his bow tie:

> Under normal conditions the necessary numerous small delicate movements had followed each other in the proper sequence almost automatically, and the act of tying when first started had proceeded without much conscious attention. Subjectively, the patient felt as if he had to stop because "his fingers did not know the next move." He had the same feeling as when one recites a poem or sings a song and gets lost. The only way is to start from the beginning. It was felt as if the delay in the succession of movements (due to paresis and spasticity) interrupted a chain of more or less automatic movements. Consciously directing attention to the finger movements did not improve the performance; on the contrary it made it quite impossible.

Excerpted from "Self-Observations and Neuro-Anatomical Considerations After a Stroke," by A. Brodal, *Brain 96* (1973), by permission of Oxford University Press.

---

a phrase. She just couldn't pick out certain words. Her therapist kept a list of these misbegotten words. On it were such simple words and phrases as "apple," "fit to print," "traffic," and "that is."

Speak only in song. Several of our patients had lost the ability to speak, but they still could sing a few songs quite clearly, those jingles that had been ingrained within their minds, such as "Happy Birthday" or "Row, Row, Row Your Boat." For these patients, our speech therapists added a "sing-song" melody to short phrases. Eventually, they were able to sing out their requests. They could sing that they wanted to use the telephone, see a friend, go to the bathroom. This strategy is called "melodic intonation."

Display symptoms of Wernicke's (fluent) aphasia. Unlike their Broca cousins, stroke patients who suffer from Wernicke's aphasia may produce many words, but they will be unable to communicate effectively. Their ability to understand language is impaired and they substitute inappropriate words, or make up new words, within their normal sentences. They may not even understand their own thoughts. This language loss frequently is seen in those patients who do not have any numbness or paralysis of their limbs.

Left-Brain Stroke Symptom Three: Depression and Anxiety

Fact: a series of studies found that up to 27 percent of stroke patients showed symptoms of a major poststroke depression with their first stroke.

Fact: an additional 15 percent to 40 percent experience symptoms of depression within two months following a stroke.

Fact: depression can eventually occur in up to 70 percent of all patients whose strokes caused damage in the left frontal lobe, but fewer patients who suffered from right-hemisphere strokes had the same diagnosis.

Fact: antidepressant medications effectively treat depression and significantly improve rehabilitation outcomes.

Poststroke depression can be the result of a loss of brain chemicals that are damaged by brain injury. It can also be a reaction to a loss of one's functional abilities.

Depression is characterized by

- persistent sadness

- appetite changes

- loss of interest in ordinary activites

- irritability

- excessive crying

- rumination

- too much or too little sleep

- withdrawal

- inability to concentrate

- loss of self-esteem

- helpless and hopeless thoughts

- suicidal ideation

In stroke, these symptoms are compounded by the physical handicaps, the language disabilities, and the other devastating characteristics of the stroke itself, which can make the biological, stroke-created depression worse. We see patients who become uncooperative in their rehabilitation. They become withdrawn; they are easily frustrated. And most difficult of all, their rehabilitation progress slows—or even goes backward.

When Mary suffered her poststroke depression, her rehabilitation team quickly noticed her change of mood, her irritability. She was put on medication to counteract its symptoms. In time, her depression faded.

Left-Brain Stroke Symptom Four: Arithmetic Difficulties

Some of us have always suffered a math block. Not so Mary. As you may recall, she earned her living by making numbers come alive. Tragically, a left-hemisphere stroke can affect our ability to use numbers. Balancing the checkbook or figuring change is no longer a simple task.

With a rehabilitation team and persistence, a person who has a stroke can relearn previously mastered skills.

Left-Brain Stroke Symptom Five: Poor Verbal Memory

It was frustrating. No doubt about it. Not only did Mary have trouble pronouncing words, but she couldn't remember things others told her. Her husband would come into the room; he'd kiss her; he'd put the flowers that he always brought in a vase. Then, settling in the guest chair, he'd begin to talk. He'd tell Mary about the neighbors, about their son's math test in college, about the trip they'd be taking to Italy once Mary was well.

Mary would nod her head. She'd smile. She was excited and listened attentively to her husband's chatter. But as soon as he left, she forgot everything he said, from the math test to the trip to Italy, from her neighbor's divorce to her husband's hello.

She remembered his flowers, the way he looked, and, by glancing at her clock, even how long he stayed. But she simply forgot everything that he said.

Along with verbal memory loss, many patients, like Mary, also experience a problem with processing information. Sometimes temporary, sometimes permanent, this impaired function creates an inability to recognize spoken cues, to organize and formulate strategies. These executive functions are associated with left frontal lobe damage.

We now have seen the most common symptoms of both right- and left-hemisphere strokes. But as we have seen in earlier chapters, there are several different types of strokes. And these different strokes can hit different areas outside of the hemispheres of the brain. The result? Different strokes—and different symptoms. Let's go over these in the next chapter.

CHAPTER 8

Different Strokes

"One minute he was here; the next, someplace else."

—Daughter of a seventy-five-year-old stroke survivor

All was ready. Jonathan had put an ice-cold diet soda on the coffee table, right next to the microwave popcorn that he'd just poured into a ceramic bowl. He dimmed the lights and closed the blinds. He settled down in his favorite chair. He aimed the remote control switch at the television. The sounds of the national anthem filled the room; the ball game had started.

Jonathan turned the volume up. "Yes!" he shouted to the air. He gobbled some popcorn. He took a long sip of soda. Albert Pujols had just come up to bat when, in the middle of the swing, Jonathan slumped in his chair, his world spinning, his face numb.

He crumpled to the floor.

That was how his wife found him when she came home. He never woke up.

A Brain Stem Stroke

Jonathan had suffered an embolic stroke that had hit his brain stem. Because of its location, his stroke affected his very survival. As we have seen in Chapter 1, the brain stem controls our basic human functions. Depending on its severity and duration, the symptoms of a brain stem stroke can vary from dizziness to coma.

Brain stem stroke symptoms include:

- ataxia, or lack of muscle coordination

- impaired swallowing

- coma or low-level consciousness

- loss of balance caused by the brain stem's connection to the cerebellum

- unstable blood pressure

- double vision

- paralysis on both sides of the body

- difficulty breathing

- nausea and vomiting

Posterior Circulation Strokes

A posterior circulation stroke affects the back part of the brain—which gets a different blood supply than the higher regions. It can cause different situations.

A posterior circulation stroke can hit three places:

1. The vertebral arteries in the neck and medulla, which can create paralysis, numbness, or breathing difficulty

2. The basilar artery system, which supplies the pons and mid-brain; it can cause double vision and balance problems

3. The posterior cerebral arteries, which supply the occipital lobes in the back of the brain, causing visual loss

A Stroke in the Cerebellum

The cerebellum, like the brain stem, controls many of our instinctive functions. It is here that reflex actions are born, where our balance and coordination find a center. A stroke here can cause such symptoms as

- slurred speech

- abnormal movements or tremors

- ataxia, or a lack of muscle coordination

- imbalance

- dizziness

- queasiness and nausea

- uncontrollable vomiting

These, then, are the different strokes that can occur. Some of their symptoms overlap. Some are unique to the stroke's locale.

But the truth is that when someone you love suffers a stroke, you don't care where or when. The specifics take second place to shock and disbelief.

Yet knowing everything about a stroke can make all the difference between an unsuccessful rehabilitation program and a successful one. Understanding what happened—and where—can help physicians determine prognosis and treatment.

In short, proper diagnosis is crucial. And, to that end, various tools can be employed to delve deeper into the cause of stroke. These are the tests that every day become more and more exact.

CHAPTER 9

Diagnostic Tools

"After my stroke, my doctor acted like a
detective, asking me this and that, probing.
At first I didn't understand what she was
doing. I even resented her. I wanted to
stop all the talk and tests and just get my
health back. Now I know they are related.
Now I know that all those questions had a
purpose: a rehabilitation program geared to
me—and my good health."

—A sixty-four-year-old lawyer who had a stroke

The year is 1890. A jowl-faced gentleman is enjoying his mut-
ton and ale at a local pub. His pipe sits nearby, an after-dinner
treat. He is laughing at something his companion is saying. They
are talking loudly; smoke fills the crowded, hot room; steam covers the small, high windows. Suddenly, without warning, the
gentleman starts to cough. He can't stop. His face turns red. His
head falls into his food.

It's a few weeks later. The gentleman is alive, but he's a stranger. He babbles. He can't move his right arm. He forgets things. The doctor calls it apoplexy. The priest calls it possession. The family is bereft. They wait for him to heal or die. As each day passes with no change, they hope for the latter.

Turn now to 1940. A different man, a salesperson, is trying to convince a customer to buy his company's widgets. He smokes, his cigarette a counterpoint to his almost nonstop sales pitch. It's no go. The salesperson, disgusted, leaves the office building and grabs some lunch at a local greasy spoon. On the way back to his car, he suddenly feels light-headed and dizzy. He collapses.

A few months later, this same man is back on the beat, putting even more hours into his workdays to make up for lost time. His doctor calls his recovery luck. His family calls it a miracle. The salesperson doesn't know what it means, but he's glad that everything is back to normal. Sitting on a stool in a different greasy spoon, he orders extra butter on his toast and lights another cigarette.

Today, we know better. Thanks to the biomedical and scientific inroads made in the past few decades, now not only can we diagnose stroke, but we can determine why it hit and where.

And even more important, unlike the stroke victim a century ago or the uninformed modern man of the 1940s, we can take steps to prevent stroke from striking—again.

The Four Questions

When someone you love falls prey to a stroke, the immediate concern is getting help. You want that person to get well. The actual mechanism of the stroke is a secondary consideration.

But as we have seen, a correct diagnosis can mean all the difference between life and death. It can help determine a successful rehabilitation program, and it can help prevent a stroke from recurring. Although you might be in the middle of a crisis situation, your hospital's team is not. They are trained to diagnose your loved one's condition and pick the correct treatment plan.

Through the use of multiple tests—plus years of knowledge and experience —correct diagnosis is, in its simplest terms, broken down into four basic elements: who, what, where, and why.

The First Question: Who

When we first see a stroke patient, we determine who he is and if there was a predisposition to the condition. This involves a detailed history, including any individual risk factors that may or may not be present: hypertension, a lifetime of smoking, diabetes, a prior TIA. If any of these are present, they can help determine who this stroke patient is.

Background clues also are helpful in coming up with a diagnosis and subsequent treatment plan. These include work habits, gender, and race.

The Second Question: What

The physician-detective also must determine exactly what happened and exactly what the event was that took place. A stroke is a general term. Physicians need to know more than "She suddenly fainted" or "He fell down in midspeech." They will ask questions to pinpoint the event in more specific terms. What was the patient doing? Did you feel your heart skip beats? Had he just complained about a headache or a numb feeling in his limbs?

Then there are the more technical questions. As we have seen, knowing the type of stroke is crucial. Did it occur from an embolism traveling from the heart? Or was it thrombotic in nature, the result of a clogged-up artery in the brain? These questions, of course, cannot be answered by the stroke patient or by his family members. These answers can only be found through various tests, which we'll be going over in the next section of this chapter.

But, in general, the more questions physicians ask, the more they can flesh out the event and the more accurately the stroke can be diagnosed. In some cases, even with good information, your doctor may not be able to determine with certainty whether an embolic or thrombotic stroke occurred.

The Third Question: Where

Where is a powerful word. As we now know, the type of stroke is one thing and its location in the brain quite another. Where is the damage? What part of the brain is involved?

In addition to sophisticated x-rays, CT scans, and MRI scans, this question also is answered through language, motor, cognitive, and emotional evaluations, which we also will be going over later in this chapter. These tests not only help determine the extent of the damage, but also the functions that still are preserved. The rehabilitation team will immediately start to build on what skills remain intact.

The Fourth Question: Why

Look beyond the surface and there's always a "why." Whether it's a family argument, an office problem, or a physical condition, understanding why something has occurred can go far in preventing it from happening again. And even more important, understanding the disease process that caused a patient's stroke also can help prevent it from recurring.

Examining who, what, where, and why will help determine the action needed—whether it is treatment with medication, surgery, or rehabilitation.

And helping in that determination are the following tools.

The Tools of the Trade

Performing a comprehensive examination is more than taking a few blood tests, some x-rays, and a cursory family history. Details are pinpointed and a treatment plan is established through a variety of diagnostic tests.

Echocardiogram, or ultrasound. A step beyond an electrocardiogram (EKG), this uses sound as a detector. It is useful for detecting the heart as a source of an embolus. A device, connected to a computer, is placed on a patient's chest or neck and bounces sounds waves off the heart's walls and the arteries of the neck. These sound-wave echoes (or ultrasound) are recorded and analyzed by the connected computer. If a blood clot is present in the heart or the carotid artery in the neck is narrowed, sound waves bouncing back to the ultrasound machinery can draw a picture of the problem. Your doctor may request a transesophageal echocardiogram (TEE) to get a better look at your heart and aorta. By painlessly swallowing a small probe, the sound waves can get closer to their desired target.

CT scan. Often this is the first test administered to obtain specific information, outlining the severity, the type, and the location of the stroke. This is particularly important in light of some of the newer "clot-busting" medicine we use to treat stroke. Although a "dry" stroke (where a plugged-up artery creates a "drought" in the brain past the blockage) may not show up for a few days, it is important to rule out bleeding in the brain before using these medications.

Gathering the Pieces

Diagnosis is not written in stone. Like most things in life, it is a process. It is more than just a series of cut-and-dried tests. A therapist will take the whole patient into account during the evaluation period. She will also concentrate on the patient's abilities, not just the deficits. During the evaluation process, a therapist will

- identify the patient's strengths and weaknesses

- establish a baseline on the patient's functional abilities

- identify adaptive equipment that might help

- identify what the patient should be able to do at this point in time

- determine appropriate goals, both short- and long-term

- determine if there are any specific abnormalities or conditions that may limit outcome and influence treatment goals

- decide on a treatment program

During the CT scan itself, a patient lies down inside what has been described as a giant white doughnut; the CT scan, hooked up to a computer, then takes sophisticated pictures of the inside of his brain, "peeling" off slices, layer after layer, of tissue.

MRI. Magnetic resonance imaging (MRI) provides a much more detailed picture of the size and location of a stroke than a basic CT scan. An MRI is, in simple terms, a superconducting magnet, creating a powerful magnetic force that, with the aid of radio frequencies, can take pictures of the brain. Because its images are based on molecular principles, an MRI is not bound by the same constrictions as a CT scan. It can take pictures of the brain past any skeletal structures; it can depict extraordinary details of specific, minute areas within the brain. An MRI can show areas of the brain that have had previous damage during a "silent" stroke. An MRI is particularly good at looking at the brain stem and cerebellum.

SPECT and PET scans. Although PET scans may sound like x-rays performed on your favorite cat or dog, both PET scans, and their "cousin" SPECT scans, are diagnostic tools that take imaging one step further. A combination of chemistry and technology, positron emission tomography (or PET) and single photon emission computed tomography (or SPECT) actually map the metabolic activity of the various chemicals in the brain via an injection of a "tagged" radioactive liquid. They take pictures of the biochemical reactions that occur in the liquid message's journey through the brain's blood vessels. Their exquisite detail actually can show the inactivity caused by a stroke.

In the future, these scans may be an excellent tool to monitor the effects of medicines on blood flow in the brain.

Angiography. This still is the test of choice for visualizing the cerebral arteries—and, subsequently, any pathological changes caused by stroke. Pictures of the blood vessels in the neck and brain are obtained in one of two ways:

1. **Magnetic resonance angiography (MRA)** is performed with an MRI machine; it safely produces pictures of the larger arteries in the brain and neck.

2. Higher-quality images are obtained with a **conventional angiogram;** it requires a liquid dye to be injected directly into the artery. Doctors can see if there is any narrowing caused by clots or lesions as the dye speeds along. Unfortunately, an angiogram is an invasive test. And there are risks. People can develop allergies from the dye that is injected to make the arteries visible. Fortunately, new technology and improved dyes have greatly decreased these risks.

FIM. More of an evaluation than an actual test, the FIM, or Functional Independence Measure, is exactly as it sounds: it measures a stroke patient's ability to function. It determines the level at which a patient can take care of himself and how well he can move around. Although it is possible for a stroke patient to be independent despite an extreme injury, the two are usually related. The more damage, the less independent a person will be.

FIM is a highly detailed assessment involving all rehabilitation disciplines. It uses eighteen categories, including

- feeding oneself

- bathing

- personal grooming

- controlling one's bowel and bladder

- dressing

- an ability to move from a chair to a bed

- walking solo or wheelchair function

- problem solving

- comprehension

- expression

Each of these categories is given a score, rating the patient on a seven-point scale from total assistance (one) to total independence (seven). FIM can draw a fairly accurate picture of a patient's functional abilities and track them through the rehabilitation process.

FIM is the most current and most reliable of the functional tests. It now is used in rehabilitation and acute care hospitals across the country.

BDAE and other language function tests. There's more to recovery than mobility and self-care, and there's more to diagnose than the purely physical. Language impairment, or aphasia, is a common symptom of stroke. Tests such as the Boston Diagnostic Aphasia Examination (BDAE) and the modified Western Aphasia Battery (WAB) help determine the extent of language—and nonlanguage—impairment. Various questions and commands analyze reading comprehension, speech fluency and abilities, auditory comprehension, repetition skills, and perception. Here's an example, taken from the standard BDAE:

> A customer walked into a hotel carrying a coil of rope in one hand and a suitcase in the other. The hotel clerk asked, "Pardon me, sir, but will you tell me what the rope is for?"
>
> "Yes," responded the man, "that's my fire escape!"
>
> "I'm sorry, sir," said the clerk, "but all guests carrying their own fire escapes must pay in advance."

- Was the customer carrying a suitcase in each hand?

- Was he carrying something unusual in one hand?

- Did the clerk trust this guest?

- Was the clerk suspicious of this guest?

Cognitive skills testing. As we also can see from this example, tests used to measure language function also measure mental capacity. But for specific memory and cognitive comprehension skills, more specific tests are needed. These include the Mini-Mental Status Exam, the Ross Memory Test, the Kahn Goldfarb Test, and the Cognitive Linguistic Screening Battery, which tests auditory and visual attention span, sequencing capability, writing skills, and even the ability to understand a joke. Here's an example from the Cognitive Linguistic Screening Battery:

> What did the ocean say to the shore?
>
> ■ I have a fish.
>
> ■ Nothing. It just waved.
>
> ■ Oceans don't talk.

Here's another example, taken from the Kahn Goldfarb Test:

> ■ What city are you in now?
>
> ■ What year is it?
>
> ■ How old are you?
>
> ■ When is your birthday?

Mood assessment. It's a fact. As we have seen, depression is a common aftermath of stroke, especially in left-hemisphere infarctions. A depression can sabotage rehabilitation; mood can affect outcome. Thus, emotions, too, must be evaluated and diagnosed. Some of these tests follow:

■ The **Beck Depression Inventory (BDI)** rates twenty-one questions in a self-reporting inventory; the way people answer measures their symptoms—if any—of depression. First introduced in 1961, the BDI takes only ten minutes to complete and requires only a fifth- or sixth-grade reading level. The questions cover specific attitudes about depression such as sadness, guilt, suicidal thoughts, and social withdrawal. The BDI is easy to administer and its universal acceptance by people involved in the health profession makes it a perfect tool to measure depression in the stroke survivor.

■ The **Zung Scale** is a self-rating depression assessment. It helps uncover "masked depression," or those conditions that hide an underlying depressive disorder.

These, then, are the tools of the trade, the diagnostic tests that help determine the severity of a stroke and the proper rehabilitation program—whether it is medication, surgery, physical and occupational therapy, or a combination of them all.

Let's now turn to these specific treatments and go to the most important aspect of a stroke's aftermath: rehabilitation.

PART III

After
the
Storm

CHAPTER 10

Coming Back: Medication

"I never thought medication would work
so well. But it has—and it does. Pure and
simple, I believe it's one of the single most
important factors for preventing a stroke
from disabling me ever again."

—*A seventy-year-old grandmother*
who had a stroke

Heparin, tPA, Plavix®, Aggrenox®, Coumadin®, even aspirin—these are the names of some of the medicines that work, that help stroke survivors recover, that help them regain normal lives, that help prevent them from developing another stroke.

Today, thanks to the advances made in neurology, pharmacology, science, and technology, medication therapy is more effective than ever. We now know the anatomy of the brain. We now know the intricate maneuvers of blood and its substances as it surges through the passageways of the body. We now know how blood coagulates—and its biological, neurological, and emotional aftermath.

To help you understand the action behind the words, we have described the most common medications used in treating stroke. But please note that the following lists are meant only as a brief introduction to medication therapy. None of these are a substitute for your doctor. Nor should any of these medications be administered without your doctor's supervision.

Clot Busters

Almost everyone today has heard of the medicine that helps dissolve blood clots in the heart's arteries and stop heart attacks dead in their tracks. But it is only since June 1996 that the clot-busting drug tPA (Tissue Plasminogen Activator) has been approved by the FDA for use in ischemic strokes. In an ideal situation, tPA dissolves the clot, blood returns to the oxygen-starved brain, and the patient's paralysis goes away. Overall, the use of tPA reversed the effects of stroke in 12 percent of patients and significantly improved functional outcomes. But there is a real downside: bleeding into the brain with worsening of the stroke occurred in patients 6 percent of the time.

Guidelines for tPA use include the following:

- Dial 911 for stroke. Time is of the essence!

- Treatment with tPA must begin within three hours of stroke onset.

- There must be no evidence of bleeding on the CT scan.

- People who have very high blood pressure, recently used blood thinners, or had a large stroke as depicted on the CT scan are not candidates for tPA.

- Giving tPA is easy. Getting the public educated—and those who have a stroke to the hospital in time—is not.

- Remember this slogan: Time is brain!

tPA isn't for everyone, but you'll never know if it will work for you unless you get to the hospital immediately.

Brand name: Activase®

Anticoagulants

It makes sense. Because most infarctions occur from clotted blood clogging an artery, a medication that can prevent blood from clotting should go far in preventing stroke. Thus, the anticoagulants were born. Although most people say these medications "thin" blood, this is not really true. Rather, anticoagulants prevent clot formation. The anticoagulant Heparin is administered through a vein directly into a blood vessel and its use is restricted to the inpatient setting. Patients may be started on Heparin in the hospital and then are switched to Coumadin®, an oral anticoagulant, for outpatient use.

Anticoagulants, however, are not without their risks. Coumadin®, for example, is actually rat poison (all the more reason you need your doctor's supervision!). Anticoagulants can cause bleeding or a serious hemorrhage and must be carefully monitored. Many medications, such as aspirin and ibuprofen, interact with Coumadin®, and regular blood tests are required for as long as it is taken.

Studies have not found anticoagulants to be effective in TIA prevention or an actual ischemic stroke. Other studies, however, have found that anticoagulants do work in embolic strokes that begin in the heart, particularly in patients with atrial fibrillation.

Coumadin® reduces the risk of stroke in atrial fibrillation patients by about two-thirds, especially if the patient is older than 65 and has other risk factors.

Brand names: Coumadin®, Heparin

Over-the-Counter Aspirin

When the rumors first began, they were scoffed at as old wives' tales. But the statistics are in and the facts are clear. Ordinary, run-of-the-mill aspirin can help:

- reduce stroke recurrence

- lessen clot formation in the blood

- decrease platelet stickiness

- prevent clot formation in the heart

In terms of numbers, studies have found that aspirin can reduce the chances of getting another stroke by 25 percent. And in those patients who have atrial fibrillation, aspirin has been found to reduce the risk of stroke, but not as effectively as Coumadin®.

Aspirin seems to work best in those patients who have had a TIA or a stroke. It can prevent additional, more severe attacks and also can decrease death from other vascular causes, such as heart attack. Many physicians will tell patients with multiple risk factors (diabetes, heart disease, high cholesterol) to take aspirin even though they have not had a stroke or TIA.

However, one serious side effect exists. Studies suggest that aspirin may increase the risk of cerebral hemorrhagic strokes, especially in those with uncontrolled high blood pressure, cerebral vascular malformation, and previous cerebral hemorrhage.

Drink to Your Health

According to various reports, drinking one glass of alcohol a day can lower stroke risk. Apparently, the alcohol content helps raise HDL, the good cholesterol that counteracts the bad, in the bloodstream.

But please note: moderation is the key. Excessive drinking increases your risk of hemorrhagic stroke.

Cheers!

As with many medications, a lower dosage may be as beneficial as a higher dose. Some clinicians recommend one low-dose aspirin (81 milligrams) daily while other doctors still recommend one regular aspirin (325 milligrams) each day.

Side effects can include nausea, bruising, and gastrointestinal bleeding.

Be sure to check with your physician before deciding on taking an aspirin every day.

Brand names: St. Joseph's®, Bufferin®, Bayer®

Antiplatelet Agents

Until recently, we only had aspirin, but now a number of new, highly effective medications have been approved to decrease platelet stickiness and prevent the formation of blood clots.

The last few years have brought remarkable progress and hope for the stroke survivor. In addition to our good old standby aspirin, the "Grande Dame" of blood clot prevention, we now have multiple medications that also decrease platelet stickiness and clot formation—and go a long way toward preventing another stroke or vascular death. One has only to turn on the television or open a magazine and you will see advertisements for these medications. That should give you an idea of how many people are candidates for some type of medicine to prevent a heart attack or stroke. Remember, heart attack is #1 and stroke is #3 when it comes to the causes of death in adults.

In the meantime, let's take a look at the two other agents:

Aggrenox® (aspirin plus long-acting dipyridamole) is a reformulation of a drug called dipyridamole that didn't work solo when tried in the past; studies found that there was no benefit to stroke patients when only dipyridamole was used. But newer studies show that when a higher dose of dipyridamole in a sustained release form is combined with aspirin, the results are much better. In fact, in some studies Aggrenox® is more effective than aspirin alone in preventing a second stroke or a stroke after a TIA. It is taken twice a day and has side effects comparable to aspirin.

Plavix® (clopidogrel) is the other major player in the field. It too works to prevent strokes by inhibiting platelet stickiness and the formation of blood clots. Taken once a day, it is also equal to or better than aspirin alone in preventing a stroke after a TIA or a recurrent stroke. In stroke patients, one should not combine it with aspirin because of the increased risk of bleeding.

Many physicians still recommend aspirin alone as the antiplatelet agent of choice because it is easy to take and inexpensive.

Aphasia Treatment

Language disorder, or aphasia, is a common symptom of stroke. Although speech and cognitive rehabilitation aid recovery, we are always looking for a drug that might help speed things along. When aphasia crops up as an inability and hesitancy to speak or as an inability to find the appropriate word, researchers have been trying drugs that work on the chemical dopamine in the brain. Results are inconclusive, but we will keep searching. . . .

Aspirin, Aggrenox® (extended-release dipyridamole), and Plavix® (clopidogrel) are all acceptable choices in the treatment of TIA, noncardiac TIA, or stroke.

How does your doctor help you make the choice between these medications? Check out the literature and talk with your physician. The decision could make a big difference in your future.

On the Horizon: Neuroprotective Agents

Remember: Time is brain—and the sooner we can find a drug that will improve the brain's ability to handle a decrease in blood flow and oxygen, the sooner we will be able to decrease the disabling effects of stroke. Several exciting new experimental agents have shown promise, but we are still a ways off from seeing any positive results in humans. Stay tuned. Good things are around the corner.

Brand names: All experimental. Not yet FDA-approved.

Antidepressants

Depression occurs commonly after stroke. Between 30 percent and 50 percent of all people who have a stroke become depressed, and, worse, they remain at increased risk for two years. This stems from two roots:

1. Stroke changes the chemical composition in the brain, leading to depression.

2. At the same time, many patients develop depression as a reaction to what they have lost: their functional abilities.

But all is not grim. Much of this problem can be treated successfully with antidepressant medication. Studies have found that these medications, such as Effexor®, Prozac®, Lexapro®, Paxil®, and Zoloft®, can significantly reduce depression in stroke patients.

Furthermore, treating a stroke patient's depression with antidepressants also has been found to enhance his physical and cognitive rehabilitation.

Each antidepressant has its own side effects, including sleep disturbances, agitation, and sexual dysfunction. Some of the older antidepressants interfere with cognition (the ability to "know") and should be avoided. A clinician must take a patient's individual stroke symptoms into account when determining which medication is best.

Our newer antidepressant medications are so effective that frequently the importance of psychology is ignored. However, both medication and counseling are important. Studies have shown that used together the result is superior to either used alone.

Brand names: Effexor®, Prozac®, Zoloft®, Paxil®, Lexapro®, Celexa®

Stimulants

When physicians mention the use of a stimulant medication, the first reaction is usually less than enthusiastic. Patients and their families picture children with attention deficit disorders or conjure up the horrors of amphetamine abuse.

But this close-minded thinking may make them miss a very important treatment both in the early and latter phases of stroke rehabilitation. According to experimental evidence, animals treated with amphetamines immediately after their stroke recover to a higher functional level. In other words, stimulants may either have a protective effect on brain cells or assist in their recovery after a stroke. This is still far from common practice in most acute care hospitals, but that can change as more research shows the effectiveness of these medications.

On the other hand, physicians do use a good deal of amphetamine-like drugs during rehabilitation. Ritalin® (methylphenidate) and the newest medication, Provigil® (modafinil), seem to improve overall alertness, attention, and concentration. When stroke survivors undergoing rehabilitation are given these medications, they show definite improvement in daytime sleepiness and fatigue—two very common problems for most stroke survivors.

These amphetamine-like drugs also have been found to increase attention and concentration in stroke survivors—improving the quality not only of rehabilitation therapy sessions, but of the patient's life as well.

Even better, these medications are exceedingly safe—even among the elderly. The main obstacles to stimulants have less to do with physical and mental benefits and more to do with their social stigma and a physician's reluctance to prescribe them. Think about it. Is it truly wrong to give an elderly patient a little Ritalin® or Provigil® if she has trouble staying awake during the day or complains of low energy levels? Absolutely not. If stimulants sound like a good solution to you, ask your doctor for more information. There's nothing to lose but lethargy and an inability to concentrate; you will know within thirty days if these medications are working.

Tranquilizers

Like their antidepressant cousins, tranquilizers can help decrease the emotional anxiety that accompanies stroke, which, if left unchecked, could sabotage the rehabilitation process.

And this anxiety is very real. The fear of a stroke recurring, the fear that it is still in progress, the overwhelming fear of how their lives will change—all these can create irritability, anxiety, and insomnia.

Tranquilizers can help ease the pain of these fears, but, as with antidepressants, they must be closely monitored. They can interfere with cognitive abilities. Their use should be "time limited" to avoid dependence.

Side effects include drowsiness, dizziness, and possible addiction.

Brand names: Valium®, Xanax®, Ativan®

Anticonvulsants

Yes, stroke survivors can have seizures, but they are not common. If someone you love suffers from seizures as a result of stroke, however, there is help. Anticonvulsants usually will control seizures. However, regular blood tests will be required to adjust the dosage. The proper levels must be present in blood in order for this medication to work. Too little and it will not be effective against seizures; too much and there is the danger of side effects—which include nausea, drowsiness, balance problems, and liver abnormalities.

Brand names: Tegretol®, Dilantin®, Depakote®, Neurontin®, Keppra®, Trileptal®

Carotid Endarterectomy

Although not a medication, it seemed best to cover this procedure in this chapter. Carotid endarterectomy is an operation that is performed when too much cholesterol has built up in the carotid artery in the neck.

Developing the skills to perform this operation has not been as difficult as deciding which patient is an appropriate candidate. Recently, a large study helped identify which patients would benefit most; the findings show that determination should be based on how much the carotid artery is narrowed and whether the person is currently experiencing any stroke symptoms. The results?

- Carotid endarterectomy significantly decreases stroke in symptomatic patients with an artery that is narrowed more than 70 percent.

- Less benefit is seen when the artery is only narrowed 50 percent to 69 percent.

- There does not appear to be any benefit to opt for surgery over medication if the narrowing of the artery is less than 50 percent.

- Patients who do not have any symptoms but have a carotid artery that is 80 percent narrowed are candidates for surgery.

Finally, if you do decide on surgery, be certain you control your surgical risks. Utilize an experienced surgeon and medical center that performs this operation on a routine basis with a low complication rate.

This completes our brief medicine guide. But there is much more. Rehabilitation is much more than "Take two tablets and call me in the morning." It covers a wide spectrum of physical, cognitive, speech, occupational, emotional, and family therapies—all working together, all, including medicine, designed to promote recovery for the patient and support for you.

Read on.

CHAPTER 11

Coming Back: Where Should Rehabilitation Take Place?

"It was never a question of whether we should do rehab or not. It was always about getting the right rehabilitation for my husband."

—*A wife of a man who had a severe stroke*

It's the call you never wanted to receive, the one you've only conjured up in your worst nightmares. Your husband had a stroke at work. He is in the Emergency Room of your local hospital. You and your children are bewildered, scared, and horribly upset. You need to know what's going on. They need answers. You all do.

Somehow, you make it through the next few days. Your husband is now in a regular room at the hospital. He is no longer in a coma; he can speak in short phrases and there are "signs of life" in his limbs. A hospital case manager makes an appointment to see you; your husband is almost ready to be released from the hospital, but he's not ready yet to come home. It's time for you and your family to make a decision about rehabilitation care.

It's an important decision, one of the most important of your life. The quality of rehabilitation care your husband receives can make all the difference between a successful recovery and unrealized potential. You have to decide quickly—too quickly. Questions swirl in your head. What kind of care does your insurance allow? Is it good enough? How do you know your husband will be in the right hands?

Real progress is dependent on always doing what is right and best for our patients. It has been proven that comprehensive rehabilitation services will:

- increase an individual's functional independence

- enhance self-esteem and quality of life

- promote the safe return to work . . . to play . . . to living

- increase the individual's chances of returning to live at home

- reduce long-term health care costs

- decrease nursing home admissions

This chapter is designed to help you make the right decision for you and your family. It will give you the facts and offer the solid information you need.

What Rehabilitation Is Not

The best way to clear the rehabilitation confusion is to begin with the myths. Dispelling the incorrect notions you *think* you know

about rehabilitation will go far in helping you get a complete—
and truthful—picture of what good rehabilitation is.

Some of the myths you've probably heard—or even believed
yourself—are:

Rehab Myth One

**"Rehabilitation is rehabilitation. All facilities are pretty
much the same."**

When injured or in pain, we want to go to the best doctor, the
best specialist, for our condition. When it comes to dental work
or orthodontics, we want to know we are in good hands. Even
outside the world of medicine, the best is something we strive for:
a restaurant to celebrate a birthday, a vacation in the sun, a car
for our family. We want to try, as much as possible, to get the best
quality for our money.

Rehabilitation is no exception. There are good rehabilitation facilities and there are bad ones—and which you choose can
make all the difference in whether or not your loved one gets the
care he needs and deserves. And, believe it or not, there are rehabilitation facilities that are better than others—at the same or
lower cost. Further, since studies have shown that the average
stroke survivor lives an additional seven and a half years, there
is no doubt that doing some "rehabilitation detective work" and
finding the right facility can have positive results!

"Secondary to dying, nursing home
placement for an older person who was
in the community is the worst possible
outcome."

—*A. M. Kramer*

Rehab Myth Two

"Therapists go by the book. They all do the same thing. It doesn't matter who you get."

True, there are certain rules, specific guidelines, that therapists must follow. Therapists must be trained and educated very carefully. They are required to receive an advanced degree in their specific area, in addition to hands-on work in the field. In short, by the time you see any of the therapists on your rehabilitation team, they have had a great deal of education and experience.

But there is more than expertise at work in rehabilitation. Some people have that extra "something," a talent that schoolbooks cannot supply. A therapist who interacts with you in a way that makes you feel secure, who motivates your loved one to try her very best, who helps and doesn't hinder—this is a rehabilitation therapist worth seeking out. A good facility will have this type of therapist on staff. It should be the unspoken credo of the entire rehabilitation team.

Rehab Myth Three

"Why do we need to spend the extra money for a rehabilitation facility? Rehabilitation in a nursing home is just as good."

Although the ads you see for nursing homes make them sound like a dream come true for the elderly—more like resorts or rehabilitation facilities than nursing homes—the reality is that they do not always ensure progress, and they may even hinder ultimate success. Changing a sign on the building from ABC Home for the Aged to ABC Rehabilitation Center doesn't change the facts.

The statistics speak for themselves: studies have found that patients in inpatient rehabilitation hospitals were *three times* more likely to be discharged home than those who went to nursing homes. Further, a study published in the *Journal of the American*

Medical Association in 1997 found that rehabilitation hospitals are more effective in treating stroke patients than nursing homes; patients were not only able to go home *three times* more frequently, but also were able to better perform the activities of daily living so necessary for reentry into the community.

Do stroke patients do as well in a skilled nursing facility as in a true rehabilitation hospital? Are they as likely to be discharged home and back to the care of their loved ones? The answer to both questions: definitely not! And there are scientific studies to prove it.

That's right: *three times* more likely to sleep in their own bed, eat with their families, and kiss their grandchildren goodnight. Knowing this, where would you or a loved one want to go if you had a stroke?

Rehab Myth Four

"My dad's stroke was so bad that rehabilitation probably won't help."

The goal of a human being is to be independent and to enjoy a life that is as productive and of good quality as possible. A person who has had a serious illness or injury is no exception. Whether it's as basic as helping a person who has had a stroke learn bladder and bowel routines so that she can maintain some level of independence and dignity, or as complex as aiding a person who has lost her memory, rehabilitation works for your loved one, your family, and you. The highest correlation of self-esteem in a person is the ability to control one's bladder and bowels. Inpatient rehabilitation facilities have entire programs to focus just on this area.

> ## Rehabilitation Matters
>
> Some Rehab Reasons:
>
> - Patients who go to nursing homes get fewer services and have poorer outcomes than those going to inpatient rehabilitation hospitals.
>
> - Stroke survivors with severe disabilities who go to an inpatient rehabilitation hospital are more likely to be discharged home than those going to a nursing home.
>
> - Going to a nursing home as opposed to a rehabilitation hospital after a stroke has been called "detrimental to patient recovery."

The Rehabilitation Setting

A jigsaw puzzle needs all its pieces for completion—but each successfully finished puzzle will reveal a different picture. There are several different types of rehabilitation facility settings, and each patient is a separate puzzle that must be put back together. Depending on your or your loved one's needs, the rehabilitation setting of choice can be:

Hospital acute care. This is the place you go to immediately after an accident or a stroke. It is the "emergency room of rehabilitation care" where you'll find an actual emergency room, an intensive care unit, and operating rooms. In an ideal world, rehabilitation starts here. A medical team performs a variety of diagnostic tests that may include a blood workup, x-rays, or brain scans. A respiratory therapist will ensure that lungs are kept clear. Other members of the rehabilitation team will provide proper positioning and movement to prevent bedsores, weakened muscles, or spasticity.

Inpatient rehabilitation hospital. This is the place for the full treatment—the full rehabilitation program. Here, your loved one works with a complete multidisciplinary rehabilitation *team* (see Chapter 12 for details on rehabilitation teams). He will re-

LOCATION! LOCATION! LOCATION!

It does make a difference. A clean, comfortable hospital with all the necessary up-to-date equipment is essential. Studies have proved that animals raised in enriched environments grow more brain cells and do better when their skills are tested. It makes sense that people exposed to enriched environments will also feel and perform better. The "Where" factor is as important as the "What."

ceive the *therapy* he needs, from cognitive to speech, from physical to psychological (see Chapter 14 for details on all the rehabilitation therapies). The team will be lead by a physician who specializes in rehabilitation medicine, and they will have access to a full complement of medical specialists to meet their needs. The process may take weeks, depending on your loved one's condition and his progress.

Day program. Think of a day program as the workplace or a school. In this type of rehabilitation program, you will receive all of the usual therapies and medical treatments with a daily "work" day that may last from four to eight hours. At day's end, the patients return home to sleep, eat, and be with their families. This is the perfect setting for the patient who still needs multiple therapies but is able to return home at night and on the weekends to be with her family.

Transitional living. This is exactly as it sounds: a transitional residence that is halfway between a rehabilitation hospital and home, sweet home. It is a place for those who have "graduated" from their rehab program, but are not yet ready to reenter their community and live at home. In this supervised setting, people work on such skills as menu preparation, group social skills, and behavior management, while continuing their rehabilitation program.

Outpatient rehabilitation. Most patients "graduate" from a full rehabilitation program and can return home. But they will, most likely, require ongoing therapy—which can be supplied on an outpatient, daytime basis at the same rehabilitation facility. This continuity can be crucial in order to maximize the gains already made. For some people, this ongoing therapy might mean a few hours of therapy a day. For others, it might mean eight hours at a time, five days a week. For others still, it might only be an hour once or twice a week, for continuing speech, occupational, or physical therapy.

Home health. Perhaps your loved one lives far from the rehabilitation center she's recently left. Or perhaps she is not able to travel to the facility for her outpatient therapy. For situations like this, there is home health care. Here, therapists will come to her, to her house. But remember: this is not like "ordering a pizza." The social interaction, teamwork, and sophisticated care your loved one can receive at a facility is a real plus—and should not be discounted. Home health should be considered as an option only if you cannot return to the rehabilitation facility for therapies.

Skilled nursing care. In many people, nursing homes conjure up places that are dark, unfeeling, and uncaring. Obviously, this is not always the case! If your loved one cannot be cared for at home and can no longer benefit from a full rehabilitation program, he may need the constant care a skilled nursing facility can supply. Nursing facilities are not true rehabilitation centers, so be certain they will meet your needs. You can use some of the same criteria you'd use for selecting a rehabilitation facility when it comes to choosing a good nursing home. Remember the stark differences between a skilled nursing facility and an inpatient rehabilitation hospital that we discussed earlier. Your preference should always be an inpatient rehabilitation hospital.

If you have ever been in the hospital, you know that glorious feeling when you walk through the door of your own home and curl up in the familiar warmth of your own bed. An inpatient rehabilitation hospital significantly increases your chances of this being a reality.

Congratulations! You've just completed the first part of your journey through the "land of rehabilitation." Hopefully, the way is somewhat clearer. You have a better idea of what rehabilitation is supposed to do; you know the different types of settings available to you.

Now it's time to meet your rehabilitation team, the players who are so vital to your loved one's health and improvement.

CHAPTER 12

Coming Back:
The Rehabilitation Team

"I didn't realize it until my husband had
his stroke, but there's a whole network
of support out there, people and places
with medical know-how, equipment,
information, and practical advice. I learned
I'm not alone."

—Wife of a fifty-five-year-old art director
who had a stroke

It wasn't going to happen to him—ever. After all, he played tennis on weekends. He stayed away from high-fat foods most of the time. He even tried biofeedback to help with his stress, which was minimal. He counted his blessings. He had money in the bank, a good job, children in college, and a wife he loved. He rarely gave much thought to doom and gloom. Life was just too short.

But one afternoon, while he was sitting at his desk in his office, the rushing in his ears began. He blacked out. When he regained consciousness, he was in the intensive care unit of a local hospital. His wife was holding his hand. Monitors stood like sentinels behind him; they bleeped rhythmically. Intravenous tubes led from his arms to a solution dangling from a metal stand.

Here was an ordinary man, fairly fit and fairly stress-free, yet even he wasn't immune to a stroke.

As he opened his eyes, the medical team gathered around him, checking his responses, determining his reactions, trying to determine the extent of injury. Over the next few days, they performed many of the diagnostic tests we described in Chapter 9, including two CT scans, an MRI, an echocardiogram, and an angiogram.

The results? This man had had an embolic cerebral infarction in the right hemisphere, which resulted in visual loss, numbness, and hemiparesis, or paralysis, on the left side of his body.

The treatment? A carefully monitored course of Heparin, followed by Coumadin® and high blood pressure medication, combined with a complete rehabilitation program involving physical, speech, and occupational therapy until he regained his strength and independence.

The prognosis was good. He had never lost control of his bladder and bowel, and he was quickly regaining movement.

As far as his family was concerned, they felt that their vigil was over as soon as he opened his eyes. But in reality, their work had just begun.

First, there is the stroke.

And then there is the rehabilitation, the way back, involving not only an entire team of rehabilitation professionals, but the family as well.

The Rehabilitation Process

Rehabilitation does not take place in a vacuum. Work performed on the lower extremities is not done without coordination of speech and other therapies. It is not a question of three weeks for physical therapy, followed by six weeks for speech, and ending with four weeks for relearning such basic skills as using a knife and fork and getting dressed.

Rather, the different areas of rehabilitation take place within the same time frame, within the same day, within a true interdisciplinary structure.

The rehabilitation team works together, implementing and reinforcing this interrelated approach. The speech therapist knows the progress a patient is making in language and cognitive therapy. The occupational therapist knows where the patient stands in activities of daily living. Each team member works in concert with the others, in communication with the others, even working side by side with the others. This makes sense: as a patient learns to use a wheelchair, he also might be learning how to make change in a supermarket. As he learns to walk from his bed to the bath, he also is learning how to shower and get dressed.

Not only are vital skills reinforced with this multidisciplinary approach, but motivation is kept strong as well. Depression, for instance, must be treated at the same time a patient's walking skills are worked on to keep the desire for progress strong.

Rehabilitation Begins in Acute Care

As soon as a stroke patient is wheeled into the acute care hospital, he is assigned a medical team. At this stage, as with the gentleman in our example earlier in this chapter, the team consists mainly of physicians and nurses. This medical team performs vital diagnostic tests to determine the severity of the stroke. They administer and monitor the medications that can stop the tide of the stroke and prevent further damage. They also check physical signs, making sure that the stroke isn't increasing in size, that new bleeding hasn't started in the brain, or that heart and lung complications don't threaten progress. In short, medical care at this stage may be concentrated on saving the patient's life.

In the acute care setting, the forms of rehabilitation are initially more passive; patients' activities may be limited by the machines, tubes, and beds they are connected to. Simple therapies start at the bedside: maintaining range of motion, preventing contractures (painful shortening of the muscles caused by immobility), and providing stimulation.

Regaining one's life begins now in the rehabilitation hospital. Each day, every day, patients get dressed, from shoes and socks to shirts and pants, to prepare for the day's work—even such seemingly limited jobs as performing range-of-motion exercises. By beginning the rehabilitation process early on, patients immediately regain some control over their lives—which decreases their anxiety and builds hope for the future.

The Rehabilitation Phenomenon

There is no set rule for rehabilitation, no one piece of data that can predict success or failure. Even with all our experience, we don't know exactly all of the mechanisms of why rehabilitation works.

The fact is, much of brain recovery is difficult to measure precisely—as is the damage that the stroke does itself. Indeed, the brain is so much a product of multiple factors—of environment, heredity, and chemistry—that it can be difficult to measure the workings of a healthy brain; equally hard is the ability to identify precisely which cells work and which do not when stroke strikes.

Happily, we do have a great deal of knowledge at our disposal.

Although the majority of spontaneous functional recovery takes place within the first three to six months, many patients continue to make progress over the entire first year, and some for even longer.

A Rehabilitation Hospital Checklist

There are fourteen elements that every rehabilitation hospital ideally offers. Before you decide to use a specific rehabilitation hospital for your loved one, make sure these are included in its program:

1. Evaluation and complete analysis of the patient's medical rehabilitation

2. Physical therapies focused on strength, endurance, and mobility

3. A concentration on activities of daily living

4. Cognitive rehabilitation that compensates and retrains for memory loss and deficits in judgment, planning, and attention

5. Speech and language therapies

6. Swallowing evaluation and treatment

7. Sexuality counseling

8. Behavior-management programs and counseling

9. Involvement with the family, as well as providing counseling for family members to help with their adjustment and stress

10. Social-skills groups and leisure-time activities

11. Community reentry

12. Access to vocational retraining

13. A case manager assigned to each patient—who remains consistently available to the family even after the hospital stay is over

14. Accessibility of the physician

The Seven Factors That Can Interfere with Successful Rehabilitation

1. A severe, persistent flaccid state in which normal muscle tension is absent and the arm or leg is completely limp

2. Marked sensory loss, especially in right-hemisphere strokes associated with neglect or denial of illness

3. The inability to swallow

4. A serious decline in cognitive ability—including speech and language difficulties and an inability to solve problems, make decisions, or concentrate on the task at hand

5. Persistent bladder or bowel incontinence

6. Serious depression not responsive to treatment

7. An absence of family support

In one study of hemiparetic patients (those paralyzed on one side of their bodies), 83 percent improved their walking abilities and 54 percent improved their abilities to feed and dress themselves during the rehabilitation process. This was echoed by other studies, which showed that rehabilitation significantly helped the majority of stroke patients with their self-care routines. Rehabilitation

- prevents and reduces life-threatening medical complications

- maintains remaining functional abilities

- maximizes the use of functional abilities as they return post-stroke

- teaches new ways to compensate for what is lost

- helps "rewire" the brain through neural plasticity

The Seven Factors That Predict Rehabilitation Success

1. A quick, spontaneous return of some voluntary muscle movement
2. No severe visual or sensory loss
3. An ability to resume swallowing and eating on one's own soon after the stroke
4. Intact cognitive ability to follow instructions
5. Bladder and bowel continence
6. Treatable depression
7. Supportive family and friends

In short, rehabilitation rebuilds lives. Rehabilitation enhances the quality of one's life after stroke. The best news: 82 percent of stroke patients return home!

The old myth that stroke victims do not survive long enough to warrant rehabilitation is dated, outmoded, and completely erroneous. Research shows that 50 percent of all stroke patients live for at least seven and a half more years—and many even longer. Even more telling are the findings that those who had rehabilitation after their strokes had better long-term quality of life.

Another rehabilitation success story: stroke patients who have had rehabilitation in a rehabilitation hospital as opposed to a nursing home have progressed from a low level of functioning to a higher one in a shorter amount of time. Why bring this to your attention? A major study in the *Journal of the American Medical Association* confirmed that if you have a managed care insurance plan, you are more likely to go to a nursing home after a stroke. And, more importantly, if you go to a nursing home, you are less likely to do as well—and three times less likely to return to your home.

Finally, rehabilitation also has been found to be cost-effective. The benefits continue for several years after hospital stay. Indeed, every dollar spent on rehabilitation saves many dollars in future medical care.

Realistic Rehabilitation

It's true that we may not be able to bring dead, parched brain cells back to life. But we can give you and your loved one back much of what has been lost. New ways to do old tasks. New ways to cope and move forward.

With this in mind, here are six goals that a good rehabilitation team can—and should—attain:

Goal One: Evaluate, Evaluate, and Evaluate Again

A stroke survivor's rehabilitation is a fluid situation with constant change. Needs must be evaluated continuously, and rehabilitation goals must reflect any change. With other conditions, taking a comprehensive history and performing an extensive physical examination might be enough. But in stroke rehabilitation, there can be several different physicians, as well as therapists, psychologists, and staff members, who need to analyze the patient according to their expertise. A sound rehabilitation plan has to take all this input into account, plus the patient's individual needs, potential, and goals.

Goal Two: Avoid Complications at All Cost

A good rehabilitation team not only helps improve a situation, but is ever watchful that it doesn't get worse. A rehabilitation team will try to prevent complications arising from skin breakdown, bladder infections, malnutrition, and pneumonia. The quality of one's medical care and the frequency of physician visits can have an enormous impact on outcome.

Goal Three: Provide a Structured, Consistent, and Secure Environment

A rehabilitation hospital provides a comforting sense of familiarity. The routines are consistent. The treatments are designed to challenge the patient's needs and abilities while setting realistic, attainable goals. And last but not least, the rehabilitation therapists are patient. They will repeat lessons over and over, consistently reinforcing them until the lessons hit home.

Goal Four: Teach Survival Strategies

A good rehabilitation team will take advantage of those functions that are still intact and use them to the maximum, teaching compensatory strategies to make up for those functions that now are silent. Flexibility is key: a therapist will suggest gestures if speech is not forthcoming. She will suggest using a notebook to put down routines and thoughts if memory is lost. She will suggest walkers, canes, or braces if strength or balance is affected.

Goal Five: Encourage and Encourage Again

Accentuate the positive. It might be a cliché, but it is the unabashed, undisputed truth underlying successful rehabilitation. A patient might not be able to work again, but he can be encouraged to use his remaining abilities to move around in a wheelchair. A patient might not be able to speak, but she can be encouraged to communicate through the use of pictures and gestures. Remember, optimism can be learned. It can be contagious and it can help make success a reality.

Goal Six: Stress Practical Activities

Theories are fine—up to a point. They help provide the foundation that function needs to translate into action. But it is the practical, everyday needs that physically get a stroke patient up and about. As we will discuss later, it takes the repetition of functional tasks to redirect brain cells and their connections. Patients must be encouraged to use their affected arms and legs. It is the day-to-day functions that will help a patient reenter the community: writing a check, going to the supermarket and buying groceries, getting dressed, and brushing one's teeth. These simple, everyday routines can do more for self-esteem, motivation, confidence, and progress than all the tests a person can create.

The Rehabilitation Players

We have discussed the results that an experienced, productive team can produce. We have analyzed the improvements that come from meeting realistic goals. But as the saying goes, a team is only as good as its individual players. Before we go on to the specific rehabilitation therapies, let's quickly look at the members of the team your rehabilitation facility may have to help make it all come together.

The rehabilitation physician. This is the leader, the physician who oversees it all: arranging medical attention, managing medication, supervising the other therapists. She may be a neurologist or internist specializing in stroke disorders or a physiatrist, a physician who specializes in rehabilitation.

The neuropsychologist. These doctors study the special relationship between the brain and behavior. They will perform the neuropsychological diagnostic tests and evaluate cognitive abilities, behavioral problems, and psychological structure. They and their staff also provide individual, family, and group therapies.

The speech therapist. This therapist evaluates and treats disabilities pertaining to language —using it, comprehending it, reading it, writing it, and producing its sounds. He also will be heavily involved in the cognitive aspects of rehabilitation. These include memory skills, abstract reasoning, decision making, attention span, and even social interaction, which helps the stroke patient rediscover the fine art of conversation. He will be the one to evaluate your swallowing abilities and work on any problems you might have with swallowing.

The physical therapist. This therapist concentrates on motor function. She will work on walking, balance and coordination, wheelchair use, strength, endurance, and posture.

The occupational therapist. Doing more than helping patients with their activities of daily living, the occupational therapist will supervise the practical routines that restore a normal life. He also will provide exercises for finger and hand control, eye-hand coordination, and more. In short, the occupational therapist teaches those functions that introduce the stroke patient back into the community.

The respiratory therapist. This therapist provides care if a patient has difficulty breathing to help ward off complications and infections like pneumonia.

The clinical dietitian. After a stroke, a patient's nutritional needs can change. Thus, the dietitian is a crucial member of the team. A loss of weight, a need for food that helps control bowel problems, instructions for a special diet to avoid swallowing difficulties—all these and more fall under her province.

The rehabilitation nurse. In addition to tending to a patient's medical needs, his personal hygiene, and bladder and bowel control, the rehabilitation nurse helps the patient reach his therapy goals when therapy is not in session. She might assist her

Golden Rules

Always visit a prospective rehabilitation facility. Trust your instincts and use your eyes. Make sure the hospital is clean and that there is sufficient physical space to handle all the different therapies. Interview the staff. Observe them. Make sure the staff is plentiful and attentive to the patients. Write your questions down before you go to the facility and ask them once you're there.

patient in practicing getting in and out of a wheelchair. She might reinforce how to eat with a knife and fork.

The vocational specialist. Independence is an important element in the rehabilitation credo, and this therapist helps a patient reach it. By evaluating previous job skills and those that can be transferred to a different line of work, he can help a stroke patient reenter the community in a more positive way. Frequently, this person comes to the hospital from an outside community agency.

The rehabilitation counselor. This person is a behavioral kingpin. He is very much involved in the emotional implications of a patient's stroke. Is the patient angry? Overly anxious? Lethargic and depressed? The rehabilitation counselor provides therapy that will treat specific behavioral problems. A good counselor also is very much involved with the family. He will work with them, offering strategies that help their loved one cope better. He will help them shape realistic, long-term goals.

The case manager. Memorize the name. As a family member, you will be in close contact with this team member. This is the person you will turn to with questions, problems, and needs. The case manager is the liaison between you and the rest of the staff, between you and your insurance company. A case manager will explain the different therapies to the entire family. She will

In The Beginning . . .

We've heard it time and again: Necessity is the mother of invention. Rehabilitation is no exception. World War II produced thousands of young people with severe disabilities, from amputations to brain injuries. Starting with nurses who performed rudimentary restorative therapy, rehabilitation evolved into what it is today.

provide the names and addresses of support groups. She will offer understanding and sensitivity. She will work with the financial issues. And most important of all, the case manager will stick by you. In the future, long after your loved one is at home, the case manager will be there when you have a question, a problem, or simply a need to talk.

These, then, are the people who may make up a rehabilitation team—the players, their approach, and their roles. But although this whole is much greater than its parts, the parts themselves are hardly insignificant. It is time to delve into the different types of therapies to help you understand each element of the treatment program that you and your loved one will be facing in the rehabilitation facility. We will go over each therapy one by one, starting with the basics: movement and physical therapy.

CHAPTER 13

Coming Back:
Physical Therapy

"The worst part of my stroke was the
dependence. No matter how hard I tried, I
couldn't get from my closet to the door, the
bed to the bathroom."

—A sixty-eight-year-old grandfather
who had a stroke

Physical therapy is a crucial component in the rehabilitation process. And it can work to restore self-reliance, self-confidence, and independence —as these examples show:

- When Jane awoke, she recognized her husband standing next to her bed. She knew he was rubbing her right leg, but only because she saw him. Her leg itself held no feeling, nothing. It was a dead weight; it belonged to someone else. But a few weeks later, after intensive exercise, she felt something. It was slight, but movement was beginning to return.

- With his physical therapist's help, Len got out of his wheelchair and onto the parallel bars, just as he'd done day after day for the last week. He had to walk from one side to the other, holding on to the bars for balance. It was a task that took him five minutes, instead of the few seconds it would take a person who had not suffered a stroke. Over and over, he did this exercise. But today it was different. Today, his therapist brought him a walker. Today, he learned that progress does come in small steps.

- When Margaret first sat down in her wheelchair, she thought all she had to do was push the wheels with her hands. Nothing to it. Wrong. She soon realized that, like driving a car, there were basics to be absorbed. She soon learned that stairs and curbs could be enemies and rain meant puddles that should be avoided whenever possible.

These people are presently undergoing physical rehabilitation—a crucial component of the recovery process. The renewed strength, mobility, and endurance that occur in physical therapy translate directly into independence. This independence, in turn, translates into feelings of self-reliance and confidence, which can only help every other aspect of rehabilitation. They can help keep motivation and hope strong.

The design of any physical therapy program is different for the different parts of the body and for the different stroke-related problems. Upper extremities, lower extremities, paralysis, spasticity—these all have their own brand of exercise and equipment. Most often, an occupational therapist will work with the upper extremities, but, in some facilities, the physical therapist will treat both the upper and lower extremities.

Depending on the locale and severity of your loved one's stroke, one or all of the different therapeutic techniques available may be utilized in the rehabilitation process.

The SEM Factor

Before we discuss the various elements involved in physical therapy, it's crucial to keep the following fact in mind: no matter what exercise or equipment is used or the severity or the locale of the stroke, the goal of stroke rehabilitation is always the same—physical independence.

This is acquired through various therapies that work on what we call the SEM factor:

- **Strength.** Stroke can make strong muscles weak. They need to be built up and toned.

- **Endurance.** A prolonged illness creates inactivity, which, in turn, reduces a person's ability to get through the day without frequent rest periods. Specific physical therapy exercises can enhance endurance and overall performance.

- **Mobility.** For full independence, a patient must learn to move about, to get around, whether by wheelchair, walker, cane, or independently.

The SEM factor is most affected by two physical results of stroke: paralysis and spasticity. Whether the stroke hits the right or left side, the upper or lower extremities, it is these two underlying conditions that most hinder physical independence and that physical therapy must address. One is an inability to move at all; the other is an imbalance of muscle tension and movement. Both create other physical problems, such as swelling (edema) or pain,

The Physical Therapy Evaluation

To perform an effective evaluation, a physical therapist must know a patient's

- cardiovascular history and status
- respiratory system condition
- nutritional status
- age and any age-related problems
- social history

but both also can benefit from various modes of therapy. Let's go over these two physical forums now.

Physical Forum One: Paralysis

A common result of stroke is hemiplegia, or paralysis, on one side of the body. This paralysis means a patient may have trouble with movement in the affected area, or that he cannot make any voluntary movements. A paralyzed stroke survivor might feel as if his body were limp or flaccid. And although he cannot move, he still might experience pain.

Temporary or minor paralysis will usually not affect rehabilitation outcome. Significant paralysis, however, can be associated with functional deficits, most likely because it is combined with other problems. One particular study found that those stroke patients with severe motor dysfunction also had problems with decision making, communication, and sensory perceptions—all of which can adversely affect rehabilitation.

Fortunately, if rehabilitation is started early, some of the damage that the stroke created in muscle tone, balance, and spasticity can be circumvented, no matter what the degree of paralysis.

Position Is Everything

Positioning is very important, especially when a loved one is paralyzed. Here are some guidelines:

- **Sitting in a chair.** The feet should be flat on the floor. The chair should be firm but comfortable for adequate support; weight should be evenly distributed on the hips.

- **Sitting in bed.** This is not recommended for long periods of time. The same principles apply as with sitting in a chair, except it is important that the head is supported and upright.

- **Lying on the unaffected side.** The patient's body should be leaning slightly forward. The arm should be extended well forward and supported by a pillow. One pillow can be used behind the head. Another can be used against the back for more comfort. The foot also should be supported by a pillow.

- **Lying on the affected side.** This is the preferable mode of position while in bed; it provides weight, which, in turn, encourages strength and muscle tone. The affected shoulder should be extended outward and forward, the palm facing up. A pillow can be placed under the unaffected leg and behind the back for comfort.

Therapy for paralysis involves the following:

- Weight-bearing exercises to normalize muscle tone. This might mean putting weights on the paralyzed foot so that the muscles do some work.

- Positioning instructions built into a routine to prevent disabling muscle joint problems, pressure sores, and edema, or swelling. A patient will learn how to sit on a chair so that both hips and buttocks have equal weight. She will change her position repeatedly during the day to avoid pressure sores.

■ Balance, relaxation, and good posture techniques to help reverse the poor muscle tone, weakness, and improper muscle communication that results in leaning too much on one side.

Physical Forum Two: Spasticity

Almost all of us have seen people with spasticity. We can see the extra effort as they try to put one foot in front of another, as they try to move an arm or hand. It is as if the body has a mind of its own, forcing arms and legs to go where they would rather not.

Spasticity is, literally, an imbalance of muscle tension, caused by a malfunctioning set of passageways in the brain that is triggered by the stroke. This malfunction causes a resistance to passive motion. For example, if a person with spasticity tries to straighten his elbow to put on his shirt, the muscles on one side of the elbow resist the movement, keeping the arm from moving in the desired direction. The result is a prolonged contraction, a tightness that can not only be extremely frustrating, but painful as well. Spasticity can make an arm or leg appear frozen.

Modern "Miracles": Botox® and Pumps

For many stroke survivors, medication and exercise still don't give them enough relief. Fortunately, we have more things in our bag of tricks. Two of these new modern "miracles" of research are Botox® and intrathecal baclofen (ITB). Unfortunately, they are both underutilized because physicians—and stroke survivors as well—are either not fully aware of their value or simply don't think to use them.

An old foe and a new friend, botulinum toxin (Botox®) can be safely injected into individual muscles of the arm or leg. Although

Physical Tension

Paralysis often is temporary. But as muscle tone and reflex action come back, a patient does not always directly achieve normal movement. He might experience spasticity—where movement is hindered by too much muscle tone, or tension.

Usually, spasticity and paralysis exist together. A patient can experience a spastic tension in her arm that causes it to bend tightly at the elbow, while, at the same time, the leg muscles push the leg out stiffly, like a board. Still another patient might find her muscles becoming spastic only when she is under stress or excited.

Spasticity is increased by anxiety, by a full bladder, by constipation, and by the seemingly insignificant pain of an ingrown toenail. Medication can help, but these other irritants must be taken into account before anything is prescribed.

The medications most effective are baclofen, tizanidine, dantrolene, and diazepam. These drugs can have side effects, including weakness and drowsiness, but most of the time they are easily managed.

Spasticity also is improved by range-of-motion exercises that concentrate on relaxing and loosening the tight, spastic muscles. These exercises are designed to

- decrease muscle tone—to improve a muscle's function

- produce proper body position—to protect limbs from injury

- prevent contractures—which are the permanent shortening of muscles around a joint that ultimately creates very limited mobility

- teach stroke survivors to work with their spasticity, learning to move or stand on a spastic leg (this prevents the possibility of too much of a decrease in tone—which can make the leg less useful)

---

derived from the same toxin that could invade grandma's canned tomatoes, this highly diluted toxin can be used safely to weaken overactive muscles, allowing spastic, clenched fingers to open.

This highly diluted toxin was first used to help people with blepharospasm (a condition involving overactive eyelids and frequent blinking). A few injections into the muscles of the eyelids and the blinking and eyelid overactivity could be controlled for three months at a time. It was only a small leap for scientists to realize that Botox® could be used safely to weaken other overactive muscles in other parts of the body—especially after a stroke.

During your recovery from a stroke, the spasticity in your hand and arm muscles may prevent you from taking full advantage of your returning strength. By weakening the overactive, spastic muscles, the returning muscles can have more range of motion; they can be furthered strengthened during the rehabilitation process as you now take full advantage of all your exercises. Or perhaps your stroke left you with a spastic, tightly clenched fist that is painful, difficult to clean, or place through the armhole of a shirt while dressing. Botox® can relax these muscles and decrease the pain. And, most important, although Botox® may not necessarily increase your ability to use your arm in this particular situation, it will absolutely increase the quality of your life.

It sounds like hi-tech sci-fi, but the procedure is really quite simple and done as an outpatient. Using a very small, fine needle the doctor pinpoints the exact overactive muscles and injects a small quantity of the clear liquid Botox®. The toxin moves a short distance and finds the place where the nerve enters the muscle and causes temporary weakness. It usually takes two to three weeks to first see any benefit. And, although this might not sound like good news, the weakness is temporary—lasting only three to five months. Why is this good news? Because during this "weak" time, your therapist can work on exercises to keep the muscles loose and more functional—building up strength in your arm every day. However, even with physical rehabilitation, some survivors may require repeated injections every three to four months. But that's not a problem: there are no serious side effects from Botox® and almost all insurance companies cover its use for these purposes.

Under the Physical Therapy Umbrella

If a loved one has had a stroke, here are some of the exercises he can expect at the rehabilitation facility:

- Stretching routines to prevent shortening of muscles and contractures

- A gradual exercise program first done without weights, then slowly having light weights, such as ankle and wrist cuffs, added

- Electrical stimulation, occasionally used, to help energize a weakened muscle and maintain muscle tone

- Aquatic therapy in a pool, where, thanks to the buoyancy of water, movement becomes easier

Botox® works best in the smaller muscles of the arms because only limited amounts can be injected at one time. The larger muscles of the legs need a much larger amount of toxin—which limits Botox®'s usefulness.

This is where intrathecal baclofen (ITB) comes into play.

ITB works best for spasticity in the lower extremities. Many survivors will need both Botox® and ITB therapy: Botox® for the small muscles of the arms and hands and ITB for their legs. A perfect fit!

When taken orally, baclofen is a medicine that, in high doses, can cause dizziness and drowsiness. In addition, baclofen is not all that effective in brain spasticity. A small titanium pump, designed and produced by the Medtronic Corporation, overcomes this problem by directly placing tiny amounts of baclofen directly in the cerebrospinal fluid. The pump is about the size of a hockey puck and fits comfortably under the skin. The rate at which it delivers the baclofen can be adjusted as often as necessary by a doctor using a computer and wand that is placed over the skin. For some patients this procedure can produce a dramatic reduction in spasticity and pain.

To find out if you or your loved one will benefit from ITB, your doctor may recommend a baclofen trial, which is also performed on an outpatient basis. A simple spinal tap is performed in the clinic, which allows a small amount of baclofen to be inserted into the spinal fluid. Over the next few hours, a nurse and physical therapist monitors you for any changes in your muscle tone. Change is good—even the slightest bit; the amount of change isn't as important as the fact that you get some response. If your spasticity decreases after the injection (as measured by a system called the Ashworth scale), you may be a candidate for implantation of an ITB pump.

ITB therapy has made a dramatic difference in many patients' lives—decreasing the overactive tone in their legs and, ultimately, allowing them to walk, better transfer from wheelchair to bed to chair, sit properly in their wheelchair, and, most importantly, be free of pain.

The pump and its battery lasts five to seven years and are easily replaced in an outpatient procedure. The average person will return to the outpatient clinic every two to three months to have the pump refilled with baclofen—which involves tapping into the pump's reservoir via a simple injection, removing any remaining medicine, and refilling your "tank" for another two to three months of travel down the road.

Although expensive, ITB therapy is also covered by insurance. It can truly make a dramatic difference in you or your loved one's functional abilities—and quality of life.

"An Exercise Primer": The Particular Needs of Our Legs, Ankles, and Feet

Obviously, the lower extremities are involved in movement, in walking from one place to another. To help patients toward the goal of independent mobility, or ambulation, they are taught a series of exercises in a physical therapy gym. The equipment includes everything from an exercise mat to parallel bars, from a swimming pool to walkers and canes. (The upper extremities are the province of the occupational therapist; you will find information on the neck, shoulders, arms, and hands in the next chapter.)

Some of the situations unique to lower extremities are as follows:

Gait and Ambulation Difficulties

What it is: Before any physical therapy begins, a patient must be evaluated. He might be asked to try to stand in the parallel bars. Often, someone who is paralyzed can still support his weight on his weakened leg; he must learn the proper sequence for walking and how to advance his paralyzed leg.

Treatment includes: range-of-motion exercises, strengthening exercises, parallel bar exercises, balance activities, and learning how to use a wheeled walker and quad (four-legged) canes.

Family members are taught: proper techniques for car transfers, and getting from one place to the next when the patient has a pass to go home—and within the family's community.

Motor Weakness, Lack of Coordination, and Contractures

What it is: Not being able to use your legs can result in additional weakness and loss of muscle tone. It also can create balance problems and a painful condition called contracture, in which the muscles in the legs, ankles, and feet are foreshortened. This can cause even more mobility problems—and pain.

Treatment includes: orthotic devices, such as shoe inserts, leg braces, and ankle supports to keep joints and muscles intact

An Exercise Primer

Range-of-motion exercises are the mainstay of the physical therapy regime. They help tone muscles, prevent painful contractures, and strengthen weakened upper and lower limbs. They are classified in stages of improvement as follows:

- **Passive range of motion.** The patient's limbs are moved by the therapist or a family member.

- **Active assistive range of motion.** The patient performs some of the exercises by himself, but he still needs someone else to guide him through the rest of the exercises.

- **Active range of motion.** The patient does all the exercises by herself.

- **Active resistive range of motion.** The patient uses weights during his exercises to enhance the workout.

and stable; range-of-motion exercises; medications for spasticity; and watching the unaffected leg. Obviously, this limb gets more of a workout during an exercise routine, which can, at times, create too much stress and strain.

Family members are taught: to make exercise a part of a daily regime. They are instructed in how to put on and remove the orthotic devices. They make sure that their loved one's positions are not promoting contractures.

Edema

What it is: The lack of movement or prolonged sitting in a wheelchair can lead to edema—swelling in the legs that can be more than uncomfortable. It can lead to phlebitis, or dangerous blood clots, which can break off and travel to the lungs.

Treatment includes: medication to reduce swelling and fluid retention, and to prevent the formation of blood clots; and the use of elastic stockings and gloves. Elevation of legs and arms also decreases swelling.

Three Prerequisites for Walking

Here are the three skills needed to begin to walk:

- **Strength.** A patient must have sufficient strength in at least one leg and in the torso. Her unaffected arm must be capable of holding on to a cane or walker. She should be able to balance herself either solo or with a cane or walker.

- **Sensation.** A patient must have adequate sensory abilities, including spatial perceptions. He must be able to tell if his leg is bent as he walks. He must have an idea of how close or far away something is.

- **Vision.** Quite simply, a patient must be able to see where she is going.

Family members are taught: proper positioning of the affected arm or leg. They are shown how to put on elastic compression garments, as well as how to check for early signs of phlebitis: pain, warmth, and swelling.

Braces and Orthotics, Shoes, and Parallel Bars and Other Tools of the Trade

A pianist needs his piano. A painter needs her paint. Similarly, all therapists need their tools to create a successful rehabilitation program. Let's briefly go over some of the tools a physical therapist needs and uses well:

Tools of the Physical World One: Braces and Orthotics

Often ankle control becomes a problem in lower-extremity weakness. A stroke survivor might have trouble walking because she can't lift her foot; the foot drags in a condition called "foot drop." She might find that her foot turns inward in a condition called "inversion" despite her desire to move it straight. She might not even be able to feel how her ankle and foot are positioned.

Avoiding Falls

A stroke patient can avoid falls by

- being certain they have been "cleared" to walk alone

- always using a brace or cane as instructed

- limiting walks in a distracting environment, such as a noisy, crowded room or a dim, unfamiliar one

- slowing down—because quick impulsive moves can lead to a loss of balance . . . and a fall

- making sure carpets are securely tacked down

- getting rid of all loose throw rugs

- using night lights for proper lighting in the dark

Because of sensory and cognitive problems, she could very well take a fall. Braces and other orthotic devices help these stroke survivors walk. The molded ankle-foot orthosis (AFO) travels up from the sole of the foot, behind the calf, to the knee. It is made of plastic and usually is individually designed to fit inside a shoe. Shoes should be purchased that are one-half size larger to accommodate the brace inside the shoe. The AFO will

- provide support for weakened muscles

- protect the ankle and the foot from trauma

- correct posture

- help in creating proper gait

Patients should periodically check their orthotic devices to make sure that these devices haven't irritated the underlying skin.

A Disorder Called Apraxia

Sometimes a person can move and feel but still not be able to do simple activities such as holding a fork, walking, or combing his hair. In other words, sometimes movement is not the only issue.

This condition is called apraxia and it often is seen in stroke survivors. Without thinking, a patient can spontaneously move one foot in front of another, but, if he thought about making this connection, he'd never move. The slightest bit of planning and it just won't work. The brain cannot coordinate the necessary steps.

However, if the patient is given a "jump start," a small amount of assistance like counting out the steps, he may walk across the room just fine.

Tools of the Physical World Two: Shoes

Braces need to be accompanied by special shoes. Basic, laced shoes that can be firmly tied over the instep are preferable. They should have at least three eyeholes. Some patients prefer Velcro closures for one-handed ease. Soles are either rubber or leather; depending on a patient's gait pattern, leather can be slippery and rubber can stick to the floor. The choice is one of individual preference.

Tools of the Physical World Three: Parallel Bars, Walkers, Canes, and Transferring Techniques

We all have seen these "bridges" that help a person relearn how to walk. Parallel bars are a physical therapist's staple. They are used to evaluate ambulation as well as provide added support in early ambulation. They are an important tool for gait recovery. As patients improve their mobility, they will move from the rails of a parallel bar to a walker or cane. A wheeled walker allows patients the ability to regain their balance and learn to advance one leg in front of the other.

A physical therapist will stress safety above all and will help his patient avoid a fall. Some of the techniques that a physical therapist will teach include the following:

Cane walking. First advance the cane, then the affected leg, and finally, the unaffected leg—always holding the cane on the "good side." The first cane that patients may use is called a large-based quad cane, and it has four legs. As improvement continues, they may be able to use a small-based quad cane and, ultimately, a standard cane.

Stair climbing. When going down a staircase, a patient should use her affected leg first, then her unaffected one. If there is a railing, she should move her hand forward first, and then step down. When a patient is going up the stairs, however, the *unaffected* leg should go first. The same holds true for curbs. You can easily remember this by thinking, "Down with the bad, up with the good."

Maneuvering over various surfaces. Tile and linoleum are easier for walking than carpets. A patient should look down and make sure that the carpet is secured, that it won't slide. Walking on grass can feel a bit strange at first; knowing this beforehand can help prevent a patient from losing her balance in surprise. The affected leg should be lifted higher on more difficult terrain. A patient should take her time. If the surface is slippery, she never should go out alone.

Keeping warm. The paralyzed side of the body will not generate heat as well as the functioning side. It should be kept warmer under layers of blankets and clothes.

Tools of the Physical World Four: The Swiss Ball

Remember that medicine ball that you tried to throw in gym class? The Swiss Ball looks exactly like one of those cumbersome toys, but it is, in reality, a serious tool. The Swiss Ball is used to help torso mobility: a patient grasps it with his arms. It also is useful for posture realignment: a patient literally sits on the ball and shifts his weight back and forth, which elongates his torso and tones his muscles. Today you see these balls in bright colors and various sizes. They are an integral part of many workout gym routines from Yoga to Pilates.

Tools of the Physical World Five: Wheelchairs

The wheelchair is a crucial piece of equipment. It can be used early on, when gait is not yet efficient, or permanently, if a patient cannot ambulate (although most stroke patients will eventually walk). A good wheelchair should be:

Safe. The frame should allow plenty of room for the patient to perform his activities while sitting in the chair. He should be able to transfer from the wheelchair to his bed without tripping. The brakes should be easy to operate and should work on any terrain.

Comfortable. In the beginning, a patient will be spending much time in her chair. It should be comfortable and it should provide good support, with a proper cushion for transfers and trunk support.

Durable. The chair should be constructed of high-quality, long-lasting materials. A patient should be able to use it without continuous servicing. It should work well on different terrain, from gravel and concrete to grass. It should maintain its efficiency in different weather conditions, from ice and snow to rain or hot sun.

Easy to maneuver. In addition to its use on different terrain in different weather conditions, the wheelchair should be designed with sufficient wheel and caster size. It should have a good ball-bearing system, and the chair should be balanced to make it easy to propel. Your chair will need to be adjusted to the way you move, either with one leg, one leg and one arm, both legs, one arm, or both arms. Limbs that do not function need to be supported.

Easy to service. Check the warranties and the guarantees. The wheelchair supplier or manufacturer should offer a reasonably priced service contract. Parts, if necessary, must be easy to get.

Adjusted to your personal requirements. A chair should be fitted to your needs for maximum comfort and safety. If you are heavy, you'll need a chair with more trunk and limb support and more safety features. If you have arthritis or heart disease, you might not be able to handle a manual chair; you might need a motorized power chair. If you are severely spastic, you'll need a chair with more trunk and limb support and more safety features.

Physical therapy is only one part of the plan. When a rehabilitation team designs a therapy program, they know that occupational, cognitive, and speech therapies all must be included. A patient with arm, shoulder, or hand problems may have to learn how to perform his activities of daily living with one hand. He may have to learn how to get dressed with one hand. He may have to learn new ways to comb his hair. He may have to relearn the steps involved in making lunch or dinner. This same patient might need to improve his eye-hand coordination. He might need to compensate for impaired sensory perception. The skills involved in all these different functions and tasks are the work of the other members of the rehabilitation team.

Let's go on to these other team players—and see exactly what they do to continue the successful rehabilitation process.

CHAPTER 14

Coming Back: Occupational, Speech, and Recreational Therapy

"I couldn't remember her name. I couldn't remember."

—A fifty-six-year-old schoolteacher who had a stroke

The physical realm is not the only one. The other major areas of rehabilitation treatment are occupational, speech, and recreational therapy. They help retrain muscles and brain passageways; they help patients cope with those conditions that can't be changed; they help promote and achieve independence. Here's proof:

- Marco prided himself on his memory skills. Put him in front of a group of people for a few minutes, and he would remember who they were and what they were wearing. He also knew an enormous amount of information about his company, all filed away in his brain. If anyone in the office needed to know something about a deal made ten years ago, about a similar problem that had been solved in the past, they went to "Mr. Computer" for the answer. But, now, after his stroke, Marco's memory was sluggish. A stroke in his left frontal and temporal lobe not only left him paralyzed on his right side, but also damaged his short-term memory. His speech pathologist was helping him regain his cognitive abilities, but it was slow going. He kept a "memory notebook" with him at all times.

- June's stroke affected her ability to handle daily routines. She remembered her name; she knew her husband and her children. But she couldn't remember how to button her blouse—or what the garment was. She'd forgotten how to make those peanut butter-and-jelly sandwiches that her kids had always craved. Both her occupational and her speech therapists worked with her on her memory and perception problems. The occupational therapist wrote down the steps to June's various routines, one-by-one, in a notebook; she and June would practice them for hours. The speech pathologist helped June with cues that would trigger her memory and her ability to perform the activities of daily living; these cues included a loaf of bread, a knife, and a buttoned-up blouse on a hanger.

- Chris knew what he wanted to say. In his mind's eye, the words were crystal clear: "How are you, doctor? I'm doing much better today, and I hope I can go home soon." But what came out of his mouth was babble, a cluster of sounds and groans. Chris was working with his speech pathologist, learning to form words again, to once again connect the words formed in his brain and the physical ability to speak them.

As these examples so starkly show, independence is more than having the ability to move from one room to another. Memory, perception, language: these arenas also can hinder re-entry into the community. The people we've just briefly described have all survived a stroke that, in one form or another, affected their ability to cope with the outside world, an ability that has less to do with the physical realm than with the cognitive. A success-ful rehabilitation program consists not only of physical therapy, but of occupational and speech therapies as well—all working together, all united in the same single goal: independence.

Let's go over these programs now.

Occupational Therapy: A Program of Daily Life

Contrary to its connotation, occupational therapy has little to do with making a good career move. Rather, occupational therapy is an all-encompassing rehabilitation program that is designed to retrain stroke survivors in memory capability, perceptual and spatial skills, movement and coordination in the upper extremi-ties, and the numerous activities of daily living.

The Particular Needs for the Neck, Shoulder, Arms, and Hands

Just as there are differences in the way a rehabilitation team ap-proaches paralysis and spasticity, there are different approaches to problems in the upper and lower extremities. Exercising and supporting a spastic arm requires a different set of techniques than those used for a paralyzed leg. Learning to use one hand to do everything from getting dressed to driving a car has a different set of instructions than those used to relearn how to walk from one room to another.

The Rehabilitation Edge

Studies have found that with a complete rehabilitation program, more than 70 percent of stroke survivors can become independent in their activities of daily living.

Upper extremity complications include the following:

Upper Extremity Complication One: Shoulder Subluxation

What it is: In subluxation, a stroke interferes with the proper alignment of the shoulder joints as well as shoulder muscle strength. The shoulder literally becomes separated from its joint because the paralyzed muscles can no longer hold it in place.

Treatment includes: range-of-motion exercises for the shoulder. Patients are taught not to catch their hands or arms in wheelchair spokes. They are trained to be careful, making sure that their arms don't fall off their lap trays, that they don't sleep on their arms, that their arms always are supported while sitting up. Their wheelchair may be fitted with an arm support or lap tray to keep the shoulder in place. If the shoulder and arm are paralyzed, a sling may be recommended for use at certain times (although, in general, we limit the use of slings because they can decrease range of motion).

Family members are taught: not to pull an affected arm while trying to position the patient in bed or in a chair. They are shown the correct ways to position their loved one in bed, in a wheelchair, and while walking with an aid.

Upper Extremity Complication Two: Complex Regional Pain Syndrome (CRPS)

What it is: Complex regional pain syndrome (CRPS) used to be called reflex sympathetic dystrophy or shoulder/hand syndrome. It can occur in a paralyzed arm after a stroke. Movement becomes very painful, especially in the shoulder, wrist, and hand. The arm and hand can become swollen and exceedingly sensitive to touch. CRPS is seen following nerve and soft tissue injuries and arm injuries. The onset of CRPS usually occurs within three months after a stroke.

Treatment includes: sympathetic nerve blocks; steroid injections; range-of-motion exercises, including slow arm swings, arm lifts, and neck twists; and limb support through splints and braces. Medications, such as amitriptyline and Lyrica®, can be very helpful in reducing the pain. Taping of the shoulder joint with Kinesiotape® is proving to be useful in selected patients.

Family members are taught: to watch out for the signs of CRPS, including pain and swelling, and to keep the paralyzed arm elevated. To prevent CRPS, family members should try to keep their loved one on a regular exercise regime and make sure that splints and braces are fastened correctly.

Tools of the Trade

Some of the "tools of the trade" used by occupational therapists for upper extremities follow:

Slings. These can be important if shoulder support is an issue. A hemi-sling is the most common. It consists of two straps that are crisscrossed along the back. Another common sling is the NDT. Here, one strap goes over the shoulder while the other goes underneath the arm, right under the armpit. The Bobath axillary roll helps with subluxation problems. It is important to limit the use of a sling so that contractures in the shoulder do not occur from lack of movement.

Splints. A stroke survivor might need a hand or wrist splint to keep the hand or wrist in a proper position, decrease any swelling or joint complications, and prevent clenched fists or other spastic contractures. These splints usually are made of hard plastic-like materials that can be easily shaped to the patient's hands, wrists, or fingers. A resting hand splint extends from the forearm to the fingertips. A cock-up splint is similar to the resting hand version, but it allows more freedom of movement for the hand. Wrist splints are designed to help position the forearm, the wrist, and the palm and fingers. The finger-spreader splint is specifically created to prevent clenched fists. It looks like a wedge made of plastic; the fingers poke through troughs similar to a glove.

Lapboards. These almost look like "TV tables," and they are designed with similar functions in mind. They are portable flat boards, made of lightweight yet sturdy material, that sit across the arms of a wheelchair. In addition to their use as a tabletop, lapboards also provide needed arm support to prevent shoulder subluxation. Instructions and orientation materials can be taped to the top of the boards.

Short-Term and Long-Term Memory Retraining

Very simply, memory is defined as the function in the brain that registers, consolidates, and, later, retrieves information. That information is selective and unique to each person. It is based on what he sees, what he reads, what he thinks. If the memory process is interrupted anywhere along this register-retrieve continuum, there may be a temporary or permanent loss.

Short-term and long-term memory depend on different circuits in the brain, which is why, depending on the stroke's locale, survivors experience different types of memory loss. Some can

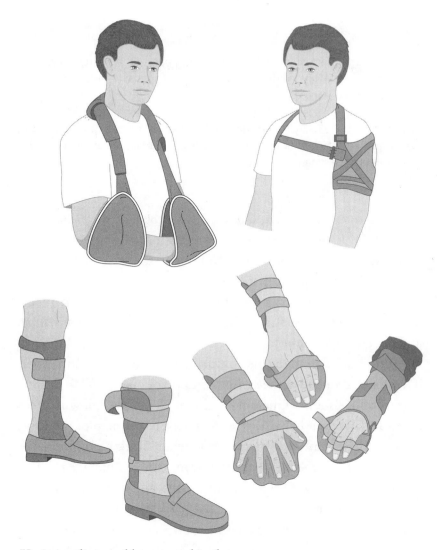

Various splints and braces used in therapy.

remember the past quite clearly, but cannot remember the name of someone they'd known only a few months. Others can remember something they did five minutes ago, but they cannot remember who their children are.

More Than Memories

When memory is lost in stroke, it becomes a part of the neurological problem: an inability to communicate, a lack of spatial or perceptual focus, a sensory impairment.

Memory loss is also linked to other cognitive and emotional disturbances that may or may not be the result of a stroke: an inability to concentrate, a lack of attention, a depression that hinders motivation—all these will have a negative influence on memory.

It is the terrible poignancy of this problem, the frustrating and hurtful forgetfulness, that, more than anything else, makes stroke so difficult on the family. Not remembering a name, not remembering a particularly memorable vacation from years back, not remembering what one ate for dinner, indeed, not remembering how to get dressed or bathe—all these point out that things and people have changed.

But it is more than this confusing change in a person. Even if a stroke's damage to the sensory, motor, or emotional functions in the brain is slight, if memory loss is at all involved, it will affect a person's independence. It is for this reason that memory retraining is so important an element in the rehabilitation program.

Memory problems, even if severe, can be managed. They can be overcome with the retraining, aid, and support of the rehabilitation team.

Memory retraining concentrates on practical solutions rather than memory improvement alone. As in all aspects of rehabilitation, there is great overlap, and speech and language pathologists will work in concert with occupational therapists on memory impairment. Some of the techniques used in therapy for memory impairment are as follows:

Memories Are Made of This

Here's an example of some memory notebook entries. It is a composite of real memory books used by our stroke patients. The entries themselves are written by the therapists; they are read later by the patients.

8:00 A.M. Susan, I came into your room and we went through our morning routine. You brushed your teeth and showered. When Bill came to see you, you showed him the flowers on your night table. He thought they were very pretty. You are doing great! We all love you. *—Margo*

8:35 A.M. Right now, you're watching the news on television and eating a bowl of cereal that you prepared yourself. You even cut up a banana. Wow, you really do love that puffed wheat! *—Josie*

10:20 A.M. You just finished physical therapy with me. You did the water exercises really great. Ten leg lifts! You even put on your bathing suit and cap without any help. *—Kristen*

Memory notebooks. These notebooks are the stroke patients' organizers, their individual "appointment books" that show them what to do and when to do it. Here are the names, descriptions, and places that are important to them. Here, too, are their daily schedules, their rehabilitation activities, and patients' progress reports. Sometimes these notebooks also will contain answers to patients' frequently asked questions. Patients are trained to refer to their notebooks whenever their memories fail them. This continual reinforcement can also sharpen the memory skills still intact.

Mnemonics. Although it sounds serious, *mnemonics* (ni mon-iks) are actually types of games. They trigger memories by associating visuals, puns, or silly slang to a word, a phrase, or a proper name. "Uncle Sam likes to eat ham" is a mnemonic; it would trigger a relative's name in a stroke survivor's mind. Picturing Hungary on a map of the world would help him think of the word *hungry* when he wanted dinner.

Coping with Sensory and Spatial Perceptual Impairments

Perception is unique to each individual. The way you view the world, what you see, how you see it, and how you make sense of it, all is yours and yours alone. But when perception is impaired, the results, ironically, become more general: not knowing your right side from your left, not recognizing where your body is in its space, not being able to recognize people or objects, not being able to see.

Unfortunately, problems with perception sometimes are overlooked early on, especially when they are combined with severe physical impairments. Perceptual dysfunction can translate into a lack of feeling and a lack of seeing, which can mean, in turn, that a stroke survivor has no recognition that, perhaps, her leg is paralyzed. This perceptual impairment might not be discovered until motor function has returned—and she's still not using that now mobile leg.

Some of the perceptual problems that can occur are as follows:

Proprioception impairment. We've all awakened at night with our arm "asleep," finding it useless until feeling came back. Stroke survivor Ruth took this one step further. She could move her arm and she knew where it was when it was in front of her. But sometimes, her arm ended up in her wheelchair spokes or in her mashed potatoes. Why? Quite simply, unless Ruth could see her arm, she didn't know where it was in space. *Proprioception* is this position sense—knowing where an arm or leg is in space. Ruth's arm can move, but without knowing where it is in space, it is of very little functional value.

Lack of tactile sensation and pain. Bill was like a child relearning not to touch a stove or an open electrical outlet—but with a painful twist. When he touched a hot stove, he couldn't feel the heat, not even when it began to burn his skin. He had to learn how to protect himself from the elements. Even though his brain did not say, "Ouch! Get away from that stove!" he had to learn to pull back his hand anyway. He had to learn how to respond in the absence of a stimulus.

Agnosia. June used a comb to brush her teeth. Mark tried to gargle with his hair gel. Susan didn't know her husband; the person who talked and smiled at her was a stranger. These people all suffered from an inability to recognize an object or a person. They could not link objects with their association; they could not connect people with their stored memory. Agnosia can be dangerous. While a stroke survivor is relearning what objects are and what they are used for, any potentially poisonous substances or harmful implements must be removed from the environment. Furthermore, the patient must be closely monitored.

Body image disturbances. Leslie turned her wheelchair to the left when she wanted to go right. Jonas tried to lace the shoes of the person sitting next to him. Linda drew a picture of herself without arms and with only one leg. Body image impairments can hinder the independence that comes from relearning the activities of daily living. It's difficult to reteach a person, for example, how to dress when he cannot differentiate right from left or when the limbs aren't recognized as his own. Constant feedback and constant drills can help re-create a proper body schema.

Neglect. Janice could describe everything in the right-hand corner of her room: her rumpled white blouse, the rocking chair with the chip on its leg, the red-and-gold comforter. But ask her to describe the objects on the left-hand side of her room and she would draw a blank. She literally couldn't see her night table, the alarm clock, the combination phone and answering machine. In other words, Janice neglected the left side of her environment. She simply couldn't perceive it. Neglect is more common in right-hemisphere strokes; it can be associated with visual damage because of stroke. Neglect can prove hazardous when body parts are ignored. For example, it can be extremely dangerous if a stroke survivor's arms are allowed to dangle precariously close to the spokes of the wheelchair.

Spatial relationship disturbance. Margaret couldn't find the white soap in the white soap dish. Larry couldn't put his key in his lock. Christine couldn't lift up her coffee mug and put it back on the table in the same place. Perceptual problems can involve the ability to judge distances, to distinguish objects, or to recognize the difference between foreground and background. Survivors who have suffered from right-hemisphere strokes are more prone to spatial problems. Their safety awareness can be impaired.

Disorientation. Elizabeth had trouble remembering the time; two hours felt like five minutes. She wasn't sure of the season, if it was snowing outside or if the summer sun was shining. Her disorientation went further: in her mind, John Kennedy still was president and Velcro and digital clocks did not exist. Stroke survivors who are disoriented often have problems perceiving the passing of time. They also can be confused about their location; they might think that they are in their home or another city when, in reality, they are at their rehabilitation center. Disoriented people may forget who they are, how old they are, and if they are married or single.

Decision-making problems. Murray tried to count out his cash to pay for dinner, but he couldn't get it right. He kept counting his bills over and over again. Ruth started to walk out of the room even though she hadn't yet thought about leaving. The ability to make decisions, to organize and plan, can be affected by a stroke. These dysfunctions can be frustrating to family members. Without the ability to make plans and to implement them, your

It Isn't Mine

Edgar looked at his left arm, but didn't know it was his. He thought it belonged to the patient in the other bed. He didn't even recognize that he had had a stroke or that anything was wrong. Edgar had **anosognosia.**

This peculiar-sounding problem occurs primarily in right-hemisphere strokes and is a form of neglect. The patient does not know that he has a problem or illness—and, like Edgar, will deny the illness completely. In its severest form, if you picked up Edgar's arm and showed it to him, asking him what it is, he would answer, "Your arm."

loved one might not be able to go back to work in the same capacity or to function independently at home. The good news is that retraining techniques can help restore some of these abilities.

The Activities of Daily Living (ADL)

Occupational therapy does not deal only with the problems of the mind, the higher thought processes, and the cognitive functions that make us individuals. A major way that independence is achieved is from the simple, ordinary routines that we take for granted. Relearning these activities of daily living (ADL) is a crucial component of occupational therapy, and a great deal of time in the rehabilitation facility is taken up with them.

The activities themselves range from the basic functions of toilet use and personal hygiene to eating and getting dressed. Because the reasons why a stroke survivor can't brush her teeth or eat her dinner vary with the type and extent of impairment, occupational therapists must work with each patient, retraining and reteaching those activities that must be mastered once again. For example, a person whose right arm is paralyzed will need to learn how to tie his shoes with one hand and to cut his food with a special "rocker knife," a curved knife that cuts with a rocking motion.

When Help Is More Than Enough

As you watch a loved one try to tie a shoe, eat a meal, or comb his hair, your first impulse might be to reach out and help. After all, it is taking him so long. He feels so frustrated. He is trying so, so hard.

Yes, of course, you could help and the tasks would be completed in no time. But help is not always the answer. The goal of rehabilitation is independence, and the only way that your loved one will regain that independence is if he learns how to do these simple tasks himself. By himself. Alone. No matter how long it takes. Remember the motto: Help do, not do for.

Some of the ADLs follow:

Using the toilet. Even the most basic, learned skills can be impaired by a stroke. It is not unusual for bladder and bowel control to be affected, especially right after the incident. The parts of the brain that control bladder and bowel function could be damaged. The urine itself could be infected, especially if a catheter is inserted. Or a person who has had a stroke might simply not be able to communicate the need to go to the bathroom. No matter what the cause, incontinence is debilitating, and bladder and bowel retraining *must* begin as soon as possible.

The good news is that most people who have had a stroke do regain control of their bladder and bowel. Relearning usually is accomplished through a combination of

- signals that the patient can use to communicate his need for assistance to get to the bathroom—fast

- a regular bowel program, including consistent bathroom time and a simple, balanced diet rich in nonconstipating foods

- an every-two-hour bathroom routine, regardless of the patient's need to urinate

You Can't Learn Too Much

Overlearning is an important tool for stroke rehabilitation. Our brain stores packets of information as "engrams," which, on cue, we are able to retrieve. When a stroke destroys or damages previously stored information, new engrams must be created (or new pathways must be found for those engrams still intact but unable to "travel"). Therapists develop these engram skills through repetitive exercises, patience, detailed explanations, consistency, and structure.

Here's an example: James's therapist read *Winnie the Pooh* out loud, over and over again. James listened; it had been a childhood favorite. Slowly, in time, the words his therapist used became clearer. Soon he could look at the book and read a paragraph here, a section there. The story began to make sense. By overlearning the passages in *Winnie the Pooh,* James was able to make the connection between words and phrases. He was able to transfer that knowledge to other printed material.

- liquid restrictions after dinner and during the night

- medications to stimulate the bladder and bowel or to help the bladder store urine

Getting dressed. From putting on a shirt to tying a shoe, the ingrained, unthinking tasks involved in getting dressed can become major obstacles when someone has had a stroke. Some general guidelines follow:

- Velcro is easier to deal with than buttons and zippers.

- Clothes should be loose and comfortable.

- With simple, solid colors, buttons and button holes will not be camouflaged by bright plaids or complicated designs. This is especially important if perception is impaired.

- Belts should be woven through the loops *before* the pants are put on.

- Front-fastening bras are easier to put on.

- Donning a shirt or blouse is easier when the person who has had a stroke sits on a chair with feet flat on the floor; the shirt should be on his lap. Leaning over, he can push the affected arm through its sleeve with his good arm. He should follow the collar around his neck with his good hand, and then push that same hand through the remaining sleeve.

- This same process works for putting on pants, but with one difference. The affected leg should be crossed over the good leg; the good arm helps push up the trouser leg. Once the pant leg is on, the legs can be uncrossed and the procedure can be followed again with the good leg.

- Adaptive devices should be encouraged, especially in the beginning. These include buttonhooks, extra-long shoehorns, and snaps instead of buttons.

- Button shirts from bottom to top to ensure proper alignment.

- A golden rule: what is put on first, comes off last.

Frequently, getting dressed is a matter of learning how to use one hand. A therapist will teach a person who has had a stroke how to open a shoe and slip in her affected foot. He will show her how to tie a shoe with one hand, using one long shoestring and tying it in a zigzag fashion. He will show her how to slip on a T-shirt and don a dress or a skirt with that one good hand.

If the problem is more cognitive than physical, a therapist will use other techniques as well. These can include memory notebooks that outline, step-by-step, the instructions for getting dressed or an altered environment that prevents overstimulation and confusion. Altering an environment can mean anything from setting up a closet to place items in specific sections to a peg wall that holds the items to be donned in order of dress. It also can mean quiet: no TV, radios, or loud conversations that would distract a stroke survivor from her task.

Grooming and performing personal hygiene. Putting on lipstick is easy if your body and mind are intact. Bathing is a great delight if you need to cool down after a long, hot, and perfectly normal day. But for a person who has had a stroke, these activities can be monumental—time-consuming, frustrating, and fraught with stress. For them, these almost instinctive routines must be relearned step by minute step. For example, taking a shower must be broken down into a sequential chain of events that a person can follow, even including those steps that a caregiver would take for granted. These steps must be performed over and over so that they can become automatic once again: turning the water on, regulating the temperature, putting a washcloth in one's hand, and even using soap after one is wet must be written down sequentially in a memory notebook and continually practiced.

The following tips will help:

- Water Piks and electric toothbrushes promote independence in dental hygiene.

- Electric shavers are better than razor blades, for obvious reasons.

- Spray deodorants will be easier to handle with one hand.

- Terry-cloth mitts can be used instead of washcloths to help facilitate bathing.

Eating. Sitting down to a meal requires more than an appetite. A person needs the ability to use a knife and fork. She has to remember the table manners that still are a part of society. She has to be able to chew and swallow her food without choking. Unfortunately, a stroke can affect all these elements, including the desire to eat.

This desire, or rather lack of it, can have an emotional root. One of the symptoms of depression is a loss of appetite, which usually will occur, at least for a short period of time, in every person with a stroke. (We'll be discussing depression and other emotional issues in the next chapter.)

The intake of food and water is one of humankind's most basic needs and pleasures—and most people want to start eating immediately. As an activity of daily living, eating would seemingly fall into the realm of occupational therapy. However, swallowing and chewing techniques are taught by a speech pathologist because they involve the same muscles used in speech and language. A therapist will observe the patient during mealtimes to determine the extent of difficulty. Sometimes new techniques are needed to help him eat with one hand, to butter a slice of bread, or to open a can. Sometimes, he will need lessons in table manners. In a feeding group, along with other patients, he will learn how to use various eating aids, including a plate guard, a rocker knife, and a swivel spoon—all of which will facilitate one-handed eating. He will learn techniques and tools to help him become independent while a therapist safely monitors him for choking, pocketing food in his cheek, or taking in too much food at a time.

Speech Therapy: Communicating in the Real World

Without the ability to communicate, it's impossible for needs to be known—or explained. Without the ability to communicate, a memory never can be shared—or nurtured. And most important, without the ability to communicate, the inroads made in the other therapies can go only so far. To achieve real independence, a stroke survivor not only needs to approach the outside world, but must communicate in it as well. And that's where speech therapy comes in.

The Language for Teaching Language Skills

When we first think of language, we think of speech. But when language is impaired by stroke, its difficulties can come in several different forms, and verbal expression is only one of them. The language difficulties caused by stroke have a general name: **aphasia.** It usually appears after a left-hemisphere stroke, and it usually is combined with right-side paralysis, numbness, or weakness. Aphasia is so common in stroke aftermath that 85,000 new cases are reported every year.

In the world of aphasia, there is a whole host of problems, including the following:

Auditory comprehension difficulty. This occurs when stroke survivors cannot understand the words that are spoken to them. This has nothing to do with their hearing apparatus. They can hear fine; they just don't understand what they hear. They might hear dog when cat is said. They might hear gog. They might hear "green sweater black" instead of "Would you like green beans tonight?" Unfortunately, there is no way of predict-

Sample Goal Logbook

Setting goals is a crucial step toward independence. Determining realistic short-term and long-term goals can go far in maintaining motivation and keeping spirits up. Here's a sample page:

June 7, 2001

Long-Term Goal:	Getting fully dressed without any aid
Short-Term Goal:	Putting blouse on properly
Planned Activities:	Walking to closet
	Choosing entire outfit
	Taking blouse off hanger
	Putting arms through sleeves
	Buttoning blouse in correct order
	Following the same procedure for the rest of the clothing

Daily Activity Log	*Done*	*To Be Done*
Walked to closet and opened it	X	
Took blouse off hanger	X	
Practiced putting arms through sleeves		X

ing which words are going to be lost or misunderstood—or when. In fact, most of the speech therapy techniques are based on the premise that a patient is learning a new language: short sentences are used, conversation is spoken slowly, one person speaks at a time, vocabulary is simple and familiar, and when a word is not understood, other words to describe it are said.

Reading comprehension problems. These occur when aphasic patients cannot understand what they see in print. She might substitute a word or add a word. He might read the word backward or delete it. She might even be able to correctly say the words she sees, but she won't understand what she just read. He might be able to understand the individual words he sees or speaks, but he won't understand the paragraph as a whole. Like the reading-comprehension format on a high school SAT test,

Automatic Versus Functional Speech

Many people can manage the automatic phrases of language just fine. They can say "Please" and "Thank you," "Yes" and "No," and "Hi" and "Bye" without any problem. These automatic phrases have been ingrained in their memory for so long that they are hard to lose.

But functional speech is a different story. Although someone who has had a stroke can seem fine when a one- or two-syllable word is used, he cannot express his thoughts, his feelings, or his opinions in a long phrase or sentence. Beyond the niceties, he can be lost.

speech pathologists and occupational therapists will use questions to help determine the extent of comprehension damage: "What was the main focus of this paragraph?" "Why did the man want to turn on the air conditioning in the third sentence?"

Visual comprehension problems. You'll find these in stroke patients who literally cannot understand what they see. Visual field impairments also include the inability to keep the eyes focused on a page. Indeed, stroke survivors sometimes will skip entire sentences or paragraphs—and not understand a thing that they read.

Inability to express and form words. David knew what he wanted. It was that rectangular object sitting in the window, resting on the ledge. He wanted it switched on because he was hot. The sweat was pouring out of him; his face was flushed. His wife was sitting next to him; she was chatting about their grandchild. She didn't notice how hot he was. David tried. He tried to point his finger at the rectangle, but his right arm was paralyzed. He tried to explain what he wanted, but he couldn't get the words out. He couldn't say "air conditioner."

But several weeks later, David was able to ask his wife to please turn on the air conditioner. He didn't do it with words. Instead, his speech pathologist showed him how to use gestures as signals. She showed him how to draw visual cues, even though he had not yet regained the ability to speak. She suggested that he keep a communication notebook at hand. And with his unaffected left hand, David was able to point to pictures that explained what was in his mind. On one particularly hot August day, he pointed to a photograph of an air conditioner he put in his book. His wife immediately understood; she put on the air conditioner. "Thanks," David pointed to a picture signal in his book with his left hand. "Thanks much."

David's problem is a common characteristic of aphasia that affects the ability to express and form words. Here are some others:

- **Anomia.** These patients have trouble identifying and naming specific objects. For example, David may not be able to name such common items as a spoon or a pen.

- **Circumlocution.** "Think of the word and you win a prize" is the premise for many a quiz show. Unfortunately, this aphasic condition is no game. Not remembering a word and using other words to make up for it can be time-consuming and frustrating. If David had had circumlocution problems, he might have said, "Could you turn on that, um, that rectangle thing with the dials that makes a, geez, some noise thing?"

- **Word substitution.** If he had had this speech impairment, David might have said, "Often turn on the table" instead of "Please turn on the air conditioner." A therapist usually will repeat the phrase—correctly. This way, a person who has had a stroke hears the phrase that he meant to say; eventually, he can parrot it back.

- **Neologisms** are the made-up words that stroke patients sometimes use. Instead of requesting that the air conditioner be turned on, David might have said, "Please put on the nee-symon." Not only would his wife have stopped in mid-sentence, not knowing what he'd said, but David himself might not even realize that he'd just used a word that belonged more in some far-off galaxy than on earth.

- **Perseverative errors** are repetitions—said over and over again. If David suffered from this aphasic problem, he'd say, "Please put on the air . . . please put on the air . . . please put on the air . . ."

- **Pragmatic deficits** are characterized by a great vocabulary, good grammar, a command of the language—and a loss of the proper "social" use of language. A stroke patient might talk too much. Her speech might be filled with illogical statements. He might not realize how inappropriate his words are. As David laboriously tries to get his air conditioner on, for example, he wouldn't be able to read the cues in other people's faces, in their gestures, or even in their words.

Aphasia rehabilitation is most effective in those people who have had a single left-hemisphere stroke, who have started a rehabilitation program within three months after the incident, and who receive speech therapy treatment on a regular basis.

Greek to Me

When a classics professor suffered a stroke, he became his own study group. To see if speech therapy helped his subsequent aphasia, he worked only on his Greek—and ignored his Latin. After three years, his reacquired Greek skills enabled him to reach professorial levels once again. But his Latin abilities remained missing.

The moral? Speech therapy works.

And the Speech Goes On

How good is speech therapy? Its pros and cons have been debated back and forth in medical journal after medical journal. But the truth is in the telling: one particular study of stroke survivors analyzed the effects of speech therapy on two equal groups. Although both groups experienced spontaneous recovery during the three months of the study, only the group who received treatment continued to progress and achieve functional independence.

In addition to aphasia, there are other language and speech difficulties that occur in stroke. These include the following:

An Inability to Use Speech Mechanisms

Remember speech therapy in school? The way that you or your buddy learned how to stop a lisp or correctly form sounds? When a stroke occurs, the same mechanisms that prevented you from forming certain words as a child are the ones affected. A person who has had a stroke can have problems using his tongue, teeth, and lips in sync; this is called **apraxia.** A stroke survivor's mouth, tongue, and throat also can become weakened, causing the slurred speech of a condition called **dysarthria.** The result of either one can stop a person from forming words, from expressing out loud what he wants to say. A speech pathologist will work directly with him, focusing on the physical nature of forming words.

Writing Impairment

Communication also involves the written word, and many stroke patients with speech difficulties also will experience writing problems. They cannot write whole paragraphs. They cannot remember all the letters of the alphabet. They cannot complete a

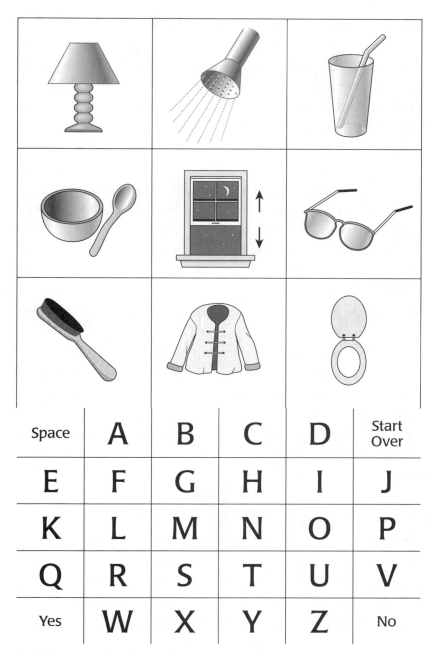

Sample picture boards used in speech therapy.

sentence. They cannot use correct grammar. The good news is that their writing skills can be relearned—or revised. One patient who'd become speech- and writing-impaired after her stroke could communicate via a technique that her therapist devised with cutout letters. The patient pointed out the letters that she needed to communicate. Her first communicated words spelled "Please help me."

As this example so poignantly illuminates, if there is a will, there is a way. Even if a patient cannot write, speech pathologists will find a way to communicate. They can use such augmentative communication devices as those that follow:

Cue cards. Literally, sometimes, one or two words will trigger the patient's memory of an entire phrase. The word "air conditioner," for instance, might help the patient say "Please turn the air conditioner on." And by pointing out the "air conditioner" card, he also is communicating his needs.

Visual cue cards. Sometimes a picture is worth a thousand words. As in the earlier example with David, a picture of an air conditioner can be used as a communication tool, signaling turn on or turn off, whatever the case may be. Similarly, a picture of various foods will help a patient plan a menu. A drawing of a sleeping person will help a patient communicate his need to sleep.

Concentration on specific skills. Although the independent pleasures of reading long passages from a book are not forgotten, the practical needs of independent life are emphasized in rehabilitation. Speech pathologists will help patients read, understand, and write their addresses and telephone numbers. They will help patients read, write, and understand computers. When cognition is intact but a patient cannot speak, speech devices can be used; she might press a button or type to get synthesized speech.

Difficulties with Swallowing

Imagine wanting an ice-cold glass of water when you are thirsty. Imagine grabbing that glass and swallowing a great gulp. Ahh. Unfortunately, many stroke patients do not have this "luxury"— thirsty or not. Their throat and mouth muscles can be weakened by the stroke; the connection between the brain and the use of these muscles can be damaged. This condition is called **dysphagia,** and it is a problem that combines elements of both speech and occupational therapy. A speech pathologist will sit with a dysphagic patient during mealtimes; she will suggest

- taking small bits of food or small sips from a glass

- chewing food thoroughly

- sitting up while eating

- eating slowly, with a pause between swallows

- eating food with a texture and consistency that is easier to swallow

Signs of Swallowing Problems

- Repeated coughing or gagging
- Eating or drinking very quickly—or too slowly
- Putting too much in the mouth at one time—or too little
- Regurgitation immediately after taking a bit of food or a sip of water
- Unconsciously squirreling pockets of food in one's cheeks
- Drooling
- Retaining food on top of the hard palate
- Poor mouth and lip closure
- Abnormal movement of the tongue
- A garglelike, "wet" voice, as if the mouth is full of water

She will also help the stroke patient: she will tilt his head forward to prevent choking, as well as check his paralyzed cheek during dinner for "pockets" of retained food.

A speech pathologist will also teach a person who has had a stroke various exercises she can do to improve the strength of the mouth and throat muscles.

At our hospitals, we treat dysphagia in a team fashion. Evaluation and management are accomplished by a team, including a physician, a speech pathologist, an occupational therapist, a nurse, and a dietitian. Even a respiratory therapist and a radiologist are involved in designing each individual program.

Recreational Therapy: Enjoyment in the Outside World

"All work and no play" might be the slogan of workaholics, but it doesn't make for a balanced life. And balance is as important for a person with a stroke as for anyone else. While learning those speech techniques and those activities of daily living, it's sometimes difficult to remember that the element of joy does not have to be dismissed.

That's where a therapeutic recreational specialist comes in. She helps supply the leisure factor while also providing much-needed instruction in community reentry.

It's crucial that patients learn to enjoy themselves again and to adapt their leisure time to their disability—to learn, for instance, how to garden or fish with adaptive equipment. Thus, the therapeutic recreational specialist will take patients to museums, to plays, and to libraries, where their activities of daily living (ADL) lessons are given practical fieldwork. She will provide music and art therapy, organize get-togethers and parties, and help stroke survivors regain the art of conversation, of listening, of meeting someone new.

Relaxation. Motivation. Confidence building. Self-respect. All these elements make up recreational therapy, and all can make the difference between an unsuccessful rehabilitation program and a successful one.

The actual recreational fieldwork varies. In our hospitals, you sometimes can smell the wonderful aroma of fresh-baked cookies in the hallways. You sometimes can help seed the gardens that flourish out back. You sometimes can see the souvenirs from the last trip decorating the windowsills. You sometimes can hear the laughter from a volleyball game. These leisure-time activities are not only enjoyable, but they also help prepare a patient for community reentry that's as stress-free as possible.

Unfortunately insurance companies do not reimburse hospitals for recreation specialists, and many hospitals are no longer able to supply these services to patients. Ask your case manager who else on the team can help with these types of recommendations.

Skills Acquisition Training (SAT): A Total Life

High SAT scores are not only for potential college students. Coined by neurologist Norman Namerow, Skills Acquisition Training is a total, functional view of rehabilitation that we use in our hospitals with much success.

SAT involves every member of the therapy team, each person involved in physical therapy, occupational therapy, and speech pathology—all of them working in concert to help a patient regain independence in the real world.

Let's face it. Problem solving doesn't take place in a vacuum. Computers can only do so much. The best way to relearn this skill is to go out there and use it. Taking a bus trip. Reading a map. Going to the bank. Taking a book out of the library. Buying lunch. Answering the telephone. All these real-life tasks can re-teach problem solving, as well as sequencing, spatial relation-ships, perception, and communication skills.

Patients are, of course, evaluated in terms of individual strengths and weaknesses. They are encouraged to pick achiev-able, realistic goals: success leads to motivation—which leads to more success. Someone with problems in decision making, per-ception, and speech, for example, will not go to the supermarket during the first SAT session. Instead, her goal over the next few weeks might be to make a list of the foods that she'll want to get in the store. Later, during the first field trip to the supermar-ket, she will be ready to pick out the groceries and make change. Success. With each met goal, confidence is built. Motivation re-mains strong and self-image is restored. The beauty of SAT lies in the fact that while these intangibles of daily life are being built, the physical and cognitive stroke-related problems are also being rehabilitated!

Indeed, the last time that we checked on David, he and his wife had gone to a department store to check out the prices of an air conditioner for their home.

Before we go on to the next chapter, there is one more crucial point to be made—over and over. The loss of speech, the inability to button a blouse, or the inability to use a knife and fork does not mean a loss of intelligence. It is a loss of function, pure and simple.

Unfortunately, the loss of function is often equated with the loss of intelligence. Society tends to falsely depreciate the value of those who are not physically whole. We are constantly work-ing to change the erroneous way people can feel and think, but emotions do come into play; they can be affected when function is off.

CHAPTER 15

Coming Back: Emotional Issues

> "My life changed overnight. All of a sudden I couldn't even go to the bathroom by myself—let alone be a husband and father. I'm better now, but, still. How could I not be depressed?"
>
> —*A forty-nine-year-old investment banker who had a stroke*

The profound and confusing feelings that stroke can create—both physical and psychological—are as vital to recognize as any other aspect of a stroke. They can make or break a rehabilitation plan. Listen:

- Mark was trying, he really was. He dutifully practiced on the parallel bars. He studied his memory book, over and over again. But if the truth were known, he felt as if he was only going through the motions. Here he was, a man who'd lived for more than half a century, a man who'd raised a family, conducted a business, and lived long and hard, suddenly unable to remember the name of his nurse, suddenly dependent on people to help him walk. He'd never admit it, but sometimes he wished that he hadn't survived. This emotional pain was worse.

■ Cynthia couldn't sleep. She'd already rung for the night nurse three times; the woman in white was losing her patience. Cynthia could tell. But these feelings were so scary; she couldn't be alone. She was afraid to fall asleep; maybe she wouldn't wake up. Maybe she'd have another stroke. Cynthia began to moan, louder and louder. It was as if someone else had control over her. She began to sweat. The anxiety was growing stronger.

■ Jonathan looked at his wife's sleeping form; her back was to him and she was curled up as far from him as possible. They had gone to bed angry—once again. He supposed she was awake, too, wondering when and if this tension would ever stop. He didn't know how to tell her. He tried but it was so difficult to put into words. It wasn't that he didn't love her. It wasn't that he didn't want to hold her. He just felt so . . . so inadequate. How could he make love when he couldn't always control his urine? How could he feel sexy when he couldn't even put on his own underwear? She'd been so patient, but time had taken its toll.

■ Milly's children were exhausted. They took turns visiting their mother in the rehabilitation center; they were encouraged by her progress. But it hurt. It really hurt to watch her, their mother, growing old, unable to do the things that she'd always done. They tried to hide their feelings from her; they didn't want to upset her. They weren't even sure what their feelings were. Anger, fear, pain—they felt all of these and more.

You can discuss the physical characteristics of stroke in matter-of-fact terms. You can detail the parts of the brain that are affected, the course that an embolism can take. You also can outline the specific points of a rehabilitation program: the exercises, the techniques, the progress.

But as the people in these examples show, emotion is not a clear-cut across-the-board matter. It is twisting and confusing, a swirl of feelings that can change from day to day, from hour to hour. And because emotion can be so painful yet hard to understand and explain, it is something most people find terrifying.

As these examples also show, however, emotions play an important role in the rehabilitation process. Indeed, the emotional mind-set of both the survivor and the caregivers can affect the final outcome. One study found that although many stroke survivors eventually resumed 76 percent of their past physical functioning levels, they only resumed 33 percent of their past social functioning levels. In other words, their socialization—their time with others, their recreational activities, and their emotional state—had not improved as much as it should. This translates into a quality of life that is much less than it could be. Another study bears this out: it found that many people initially don't think life is worth living after a stroke.

It doesn't have to be this way. Emotions are merely another aspect of stroke and its rehabilitation. Understanding the emotional process after stroke can help you control it. It can help ease the fear and enhance rehabilitation success.

Let's go over some of the emotional issues of stroke one by one, beginning with the shock, the disbelief, and the anger, which are a part of . . .

The Grieving Process

Psychologist Elisabeth Kübler-Ross first delineated her landmark six stages of grief in a discussion of terminal illness. But she could very well have applied them to stroke survival. There are six stages of emotion that both the stroke survivor and the family may go through after a stroke "comes to their house."

Stage One: Denial. The shock of a stroke has a purpose: it hides the personal losses and the changes that eventually will come. During this time in the acute care hospital, families often can feel a sense of unreality, a sense that this could not be happening to them. The same holds true for the stroke survivors themselves. They cannot believe that things have changed, that an infarction has so quickly altered their lives. They even can deny that the incident ever occurred.

Stage Two: Anger. As the shock of the stroke wears off, anger sets in. "I can't believe this happened to me! It's not fair!" This stage can have a mixture of denial as well, a feeling that "Hey, by next spring, I'll be as good as new!" The family, too, will feel anger at their new circumstances. Once the situation is no longer life-threatening, these other emotions come into play.

Stage Three: Bargaining. The shock is wearing off. The rehabilitation process has begun. The stroke survivor hopes for a new start, a miracle. "Dear God, if only I can use my arm again, I will do good work for the rest of my life." The family, too, makes their own bargains with God, hoping against unrealistic hope that things will go back to the way they were.

Stage Four: Depression. Reality sets in. Your loved one may never be the same. Your life may never be the same. Your family structure may stay irrevocably different. The old self, your old image, must be mourned. Family members might feel that they would have preferred death to this "new" person, which, in turn, creates guilt and depression. In fact, depression is so important an issue in stroke that we'll be discussing it later in this chapter.

Stage Five: Acceptance. It is only when these feelings of depression, of guilt and anger, are dealt with that acceptance and healing can begin. Acceptance is based in the rational realm; it is knowing that things will be different, but that they still can work. Rehabilitation is in full swing and motivation is improving.

Stage Six: Hope. From the depths of despair comes hope. Not the unrealistic hope that a loved one will be as she once was, that all things will be as they once were, but a real hope, a valid hope that states, "There is value in who I am. I am alive. Together, we will reach the limits that we can reach."

Not everyone goes through these six stages of emotions, and not everyone goes through them in the same order. But, in general, the grieving process, from the first shock to final acceptance, evolves during the rehabilitation process.

The Stroke Dynamic: Families in Crisis

Here's a compelling example of the emotional upheaval a stroke creates within families. One of our patients, a seventy-two-year-old stroke survivor, had successfully completed his rehabilitation within eight months. He functioned well—physically, cognitively, and socially. The FIM score, which measures a stroke patient's ability to function (see Chapter 9, "Diagnostic Tools"), showed him to be fully independent, with the help of a cane and a few dressing aids. But as soon as he went home, he regressed. Suddenly, his memory lapsed. He had no energy. He needed his family to do almost everything, from getting him glasses of water in the middle of the night to dressing him in shirts and pants in the morning. Unfortunately, the more he asked for help, the more his family resented him. It became a vicious cycle. Confusion,

On the Lighter Side

The popular TV show *Frasier* even used Elisabeth Kübler-Ross's six stages of grief in its first show of the 1998–1999 season, as Frasier grappled with losing his job the season before. His emotions ran the full gamut—from denying the fact that he was fired to finally accepting the fact that he had to find something new—and knowing he would.

anger, and hostility reigned at home, until his rehabilitation facility intervened during follow-up. The rehabilitation team helped the family recognize the dynamics that were coming into play; they helped the family realize that each member, including the loved one who had had a stroke, exacerbated the situation, keeping the destructive cycle alive.

Yes, family dynamics do change when a stroke occurs. There is no question about it. And the family's role, each individual's feelings and limitations, is a crucial element in that dynamic. Think of it.

There may be a role change or reversal, the spouse acting as a parent, a parent becoming the child.

Acute dependency comes into play, even if it's just to drive the family member who had a stroke a few short blocks to do some errands.

There's the constant tension surrounding the unvoiced question, "What if it happens again?"

But as difficult as these situations are, it's crucial that they do not interfere with the rehabilitation progress. In this example, the stroke survivor's regression affected the family and the family's resentment affected him. He became a child who could not function independently, supporting the proven fact that a person who has had a stroke must be treated as an adult or he will regress—and progress will erode.

Stroke survivor and family are linked—by their grief, their attitudes, and their pressures. Their reactions might be different, their emotions might feed on each other, but every family member must work together to shape effective strategies for change—and create a healthy home.

In fact, family matters are so crucial to a stroke patient's health—and to the health of each family member—that we will be discussing them separately in depth in the next chapter.

But this chapter belongs solely to the person who has had a stroke: his emotional state, his emotional progress, his emotional rehabilitation.

And above all, the number-one emotion that affects all stroke patients to a greater or lesser extent is . . .

Depression

A crucial fact: it's very normal to be depressed after a stroke. Indeed, between 30 percent and 50 percent of all stroke survivors experience depression. It makes sense.

First of all, there are the disabilities themselves, the very real fact that a person who has had a stroke cannot, for example, dress himself or remember names and dates. The more debilitating the stroke's aftermath, the more depressed a patient might become.

Then there is the damage done to the brain itself, the chemistry that is imbalanced, the signals that are not getting connected. In fact, studies show that strokes in the left hemisphere create more major depressive illnesses than strokes in the right hemisphere.

But whatever the actual trigger, depression can create emotional ups and downs that can be extremely unsettling to a family. It also can cause a variety of behavioral problems, from inappropriate hostility to heightened withdrawal.

A rehabilitation team understands that the emotional component is crucial for strong motivation and continued progress. One or all of the team members may recognize the signs of depression and recommend counseling. Your doctor may add an antidepressant medication to take on a daily basis.

Here are some of the emotional issues that the team looks for, those mind-sets taken root in a stroke survivor that can create—and maintain—a depression:

A focus on the hopes, dreams, and wishes that now are forever altered. She no longer can play golf. She no longer can knit. She no longer can read for long periods of time. She no longer can dream about going to Paris.

An overwhelming fear of aging, death, and the loss of independence. Perhaps he has weathered this stroke, but what about the next one and the next one after that? And how will he pay the bills?

An altered self-image. Physically, she is a different person. Whether in a wheelchair or not, she looks in the mirror and sees a person with a disability and it hurts.

A loss of self-esteem. All these elements result in a lowered self-image, a drop in self-respect. Rehabilitation facilities try to circumvent these problems by encouraging their patients to wear street clothes, as opposed to hospital gowns and slippers. Women are encouraged to put on makeup. Grooming and personal hygiene are essential. Not only do these routines help in ADL retraining, but they help the patients' sense of self, their sense of self-esteem, and their sense of control over their environment.

Depression can do more than hinder motivation and create family havoc. It can derail rehabilitation success. Studies have found that once depression is in place, functional abilities are reduced. Other studies have found that depressed patients remain the most impaired and have a worse prognosis. There is so strong

The Symptoms of Depression

1. Excessive fatigue and low energy

2. Excessive crying

3. Withdrawal from others

4. Boredom and indifference—to people and activities

5. Inability to concentrate or make decisions

6. Complaints of physical ailments with no physical roots

7. Too much or too little sleep

8. Too much or too little appetite

9. Excessive anxiety

10. Excessive irritability

11. Irrational feelings of guilt and worthlessness

12. Depressed mood and diminished pleasure in most activities

13. Recurring thoughts of suicide and death

   If your loved one exhibits five or more of these symptoms every day for a period longer than a few weeks, it's possible that she is suffering from major poststroke depression, and it's imperative that you discuss the situation with her physician immediately. These symptoms can signal a depression that, left unchecked, could sabotage rehabilitation—and your loved one's quality of life.

a correlation between depression and functional abilities that if a patient is not progressing as fast as we expect, it is a red flag that the patient may be depressed.

   But there is good news. Once depression is diagnosed, it can be treated, and that treatment includes antidepressant medication (which we detail in Chapter 10), individual therapy, and group-support sessions. Some of the rehabilitation team's techniques also include the following:

More About Depression

Many people who develop depression after stroke have the same chemical imbalances in their brain as severely depressed persons who have not had a stroke. Their psychological problems are similar. Drug or alcohol abuse, for example, may be associated with a stroke, but that same abuse is also a common symptom of non–stroke-related depression.

Depression can affect our ability to think and remember, our ability to pay attention and concentrate, and our ability to solve problems—and it may appear as if a person is brain-injured when he is not.

Scheduled activities. A filled calendar can provide order when feelings are overwhelming. A busy routine can give a depressed patient a purpose.

Setting goals. Realistic short-term and long-term goals can go far to provide motivation and increase positive attitudes. As goals are met, the stroke patient can begin to feel better about himself.

Extracurricular activities. The benefits of recreational activities are a vital antidote for depression. Taking field trips and day trips and performing the activities of daily life surrounded by other people, for instance, in a supermarket or a bank, can help put things in perspective.

Knowledge. In knowledge, there is strength. If you learn everything you can about stroke and about depression, it can help shed light on those unknown "monsters" that threaten to overwhelm you.

Self-awareness training. At our hospitals, we have actual training areas that we use for our patients. These areas hold a bed, furniture, a complete kitchen, even a bathroom. This setting enables a patient and her team to focus on self-awareness. It helps her work on the skills necessary for the "real world" under the safe, close supervision of an experienced staff. And the more the stroke patient succeeds in, say, making her bed, fixing a sandwich, or sweeping the floor, the more her confidence will build. Her depression will lessen. Her family, too, will begin to feel more able to handle things when she comes home. They, too, will have their confidence bolstered. Best of all, self-awareness training spurs motivation, ultimately giving the patient a sense of urgency, a push to get on with rehabilitation.

Sex and the Stroke Patient

Although it's a vital issue, sex sometimes doesn't get as much attention in rehabilitation as it should. As common as sexual problems can be after a stroke, they often are overlooked. Embarrassment, fear, anxiety—all these can stop a stroke patient or his spouse from speaking out, especially if this subject is not first broached by the rehabilitation team.

Yes, sexual dysfunction is common after a stroke. But dysfunction does not imply disinterest. One study found that although there was a 60 percent drop in sexual activity after a stroke, interest only dropped 14 percent!

You and your loved one are not alone with your sexual doubts and fears. There is good news: new medications and treatments can help restore sexual function. Even more reassuring, research has discovered that sex can safely resume shortly after a stroke, although it is always best to check with your doctor.

The main issues creating sexual conflict in the stroke patient are as follows:

Fear. The survivor is afraid that the stroke will happen again—while in the midst of intimacy. The more fear, the more anxiety, all of which translate into dysfunction. Yet, studies show that this fear is ungrounded. If you can perform normal daily

Emotional Outlet

There is one crucial connection between stroke and emotion: any personality problems in place *before* a stroke can become exaggerated after the stroke. If a survivor had been anxious before his stroke, he might be more so in its aftermath. The same goes for depression, emotional ups and downs, hostility, and sexual dysfunction.

activities, you can perform sex. Blood pressure is elevated about the same in both situations.

An outgrowth of a stroke impairment. An inability to speak, memory problems, perception difficulties, paralysis, and a loss of touch, sight, or sound—these all can interfere in sexual activities, especially as performed before the stroke. Giving and receiving pleasure, however, can take many forms. If an impairment or disability is stopping your ability to enjoy sex, it's crucial that you and your loved one discuss it not only with each other, but with your physician as well. Trying different positions, using vibrators, and researching and then utilizing some of the new inroads to help achieve erection (such as Viagra®, Cialis®, Levitra®) can all enhance sexual pleasure. Be sure to check with your primary physician as some patients cannot take medications for erectile dysfuction.

Emotional impairment. Impotence can also arise from depression or from a personality change. A poor self-image also can translate into a disinterest in sex. If this is a problem, talk to your physician or rehabilitation team member; she is there to help.

Incontinence. Obviously, bladder or bowel problems can translate into awkwardness during sex. This also can hurt self-image and, at the same time, the desire for sex. But catheters and other devices can be worked with during sexual activity.

Sex and Aging

People with disabilities, including stroke survivors, and the elderly are frequently viewed as being asexual. Nothing could be further from the truth. Sometimes all that is lacking is a partner! A 1998 survey from the National Council on the Aging found that half of the Americans over sixty enjoy sexual relations at least once every month. Further, 74 percent of the men and 70 percent of the women were emotionally satisfied with their relations—and 43 percent felt that sex was as good now as it was when they were young.

Counselors can provide insights into giving and receiving pleasure despite physical impairments.

Medical considerations. Many medications, including antidepressants, can affect sexuality. Make sure that you know the possible side effects of the medications that you or your loved one is taking.

One final point: a stroke does not automatically translate into sexual dysfunction. In fact, sexual problems do not exist for many stroke survivors and their families. Between 20 percent and 25 percent of all stroke survivors and their loved ones actually report an *increase* in sexual activity. In short, closeness before will translate into closeness after the stroke.

Other Behaviors, Other Lives

Depression and lack of libido are only a few of the conditions that can result in emotional sabotage. Here are some others:

Short attention span. Margo couldn't talk to her fellow patients for more than five minutes. Jim couldn't read more than a paragraph or two of a magazine. A short attention span is a problem that can result from cognitive impairments caused by stroke, and it can be particularly unsettling to the family. Stroke survivors might repeat tasks again and again. They might act like children, unable to sit still. They might be able to spend only a few minutes reading a magazine or even watching television.

Anxiety disorders. Lizbeth woke up in the middle of the night, her heart pounding, her mouth dry. She felt as if she were having another stroke, even though she'd just received a clean bill of health. Jonathan refused to get out of bed, morning, noon, and night. He was terrified; his heartbeat was rapid. These two people are victims of anxiety, a result of the overwhelming fear that stroke may bring in its aftermath—of the condition that, in a momentary flash, changes one's life. This anxiety can be long lasting; it is exacerbated by overstimulation, impatience, and over-tiredness, which can occur if a rehabilitation team is not attuned to the problem.

Anxiety can be decreased with a simple, but effective, technique: decision making. Giving the stroke patient the power to make decisions can help him control his destiny. Even a small degree of control can ease anxiety's stress.

Emotional ups and downs. Milton was calm only moments before. Now he is screaming at the top of his lungs. June can't stop crying, but only minutes before she was laughing with the staff. A stroke changes personalities; it can make people labile. From day to day, from hour to hour, the mood of a person who has had a stroke can change in a flash. This can be difficult on the family who does not understand the underlying cause. Although an abrupt personality change is not a setback, it may be viewed as such and it can create discouragement within the family sphere. Mood fluctuation is common after a stroke and usually improves with time. It is vital families are taught that in these situations, it is the personality at work, not the unraveling of the good work itself.

Irrational Beliefs

The basis for most of the stress in our lives is the way we see the world and interpret individual events. What do we believe? The clinical psychologist Albert Ellis teaches us that many of our beliefs are irrational, and setting unrealistic goals or expectations will lead to stress.

Dr. Ellis tells us to avoid the "shoulds, musts, and have to's" of life. It is rarely helpful to beat yourself up with "I should have done this . . . I must have done that. . . . " Especially after a stroke!

Abandon those irrational beliefs. Set realistic personal goals and you will find your stress levels dropping.

Managing Behavior

Whether it's anger, tears, or hostility, unpredictable behavior can take a toll on the family. It also can affect a stroke patient's success in the outside world: going back to work, going to social events, being a part of the community—all these can be hampered.

We have an expression we use in our hospitals with patients who are suddenly faced with a life-altering injury or illness. We tell them "we know it's not as if you called up a department store and ordered a stroke." But the stroke is a reality, one that must be faced—especially by the stroke patient. Only he can provide the perseverance, the driving force, the determination to help himself. It's a difficult realization to truly accept, but one that is necessary for emotional adjustment—and effective rehabilitation. The patient has to be as much an active participant as his family members and the entire rehabilitation team.

The various therapies in the rehabilitation process help strengthen emotional stability through education, self-awareness, and medication. All of them working in unison toward common realistic goals help decrease the possibilities of anxiety, depression, alcohol and drug abuse, and dependency—while, at the

Learned Optimism: Seeing the Glass as Half-Full

We've all met them. The people who never have anything nice to say about anyone else, who always see the worst of every situation. If you are not careful, they can deplete you of your energies and infect you with their attitudes.

Optimism can be learned. People with a positive outlook on life, who see the cup as half-full rather than half-empty, are healthier and more successful. This is especially true when it comes to rehabilitation. If, despite your stroke, your disability, you diligently work every day on being more optimistic and positive, you will see it transfer to those around you.

same time, these sound goals also create self-confidence, hope, and strong motivation to improve.

Added to this rehabilitation "mix" is behavior-management therapy, which the different staff members all use. Whether implemented in physical, speech, or occupational therapy, behavior management helps rein in negative emotion and inappropriate behavior:

Immediate feedback. A rehabilitation staff member is trained to quickly intervene if a patient has an outburst or becomes threatening. Slowly, without force or punishment, the staff member will distract and calm the patient; later, after the incident has passed, he will attempt to modify the behavior.

Reward system. Socially acceptable behavior should be rewarded. To encourage positive behavior, rehabilitation staff members are trained to catch patients in the act of doing something well—and offer them a reward. Every time a patient uses restraint instead of tears, logic instead of tantrums, he receives positive reinforcement. Although this might sound simplistic, it isn't. It really works—helping to motivate and guide patients back to their old socially acceptable roles. Poor behavior is ignored, not punished. Good behavior is reinforced.

Self-monitoring techniques. Joan uses a daily log to monitor herself. Every time she stops herself from screaming, she puts an X in the "appropriate behavior" column. Every time she gives in and yells, she puts an X in the "inappropriate behavior" column. The more Xs she gives herself in the "appropriate behavior" column, the more it means that she is thinking before she acts— and the more rewards she receives.

Negotiation. During speech therapy, it can keep a patient going for an extra ten minutes. During physical therapy, it can make the difference between walking a few paces on the parallel bars or standing still. What is *it*? It is the same type of negotiation that you might engage in with your child: ten more minutes and you'll get a reward. And it works.

Decrease the distraction. All John has to do is look at the other patients and he becomes tense. Beatrice can't cope with too many conversations going at once in the dining room. Sam cannot bear making a decision. Just as a student needs to turn down the rock music to study for a midterm, stroke patients may need less stimuli to focus on the task at hand. Too much stimulation can be overwhelming. Situations that make a patient uncomfortable can become overwhelming; he can become anxious and lose control. To avoid triggering inappropriate behavior, the stimuli at a hospital can be adjusted; uncomfortable situations can be avoided until the patient is ready to tackle them.

Support groups. Realizing that you are not alone, that there are others in exactly the same situation, can ease the pain and the fear more than anything else. Other people do understand. Other people are going through the same experience. They feel the same pain. In support-group settings, patients can share their feelings without risk. They don't have to censor their emotions as they might do with their families. And as an added plus, they receive empathy, understanding, instant feedback, and practical advice from others who have walked in their shoes.

CHAPTER 16

Coming Back: Neural Plasticity— A New Road of Recovery

"At first my left arm seemed to be improving rapidly, but then I seemed to reach a plateau. My therapist suggested we try a new form of exercise called constraint therapy. In two weeks I was off my plateau and making real progress again."

—*A fifty-eight-year-old man and Encompass Health outpatient who had suffered a stroke six months earlier*

In a laboratory at the University of Texas in Houston, Dr. Randolph J. Nudo and a group of monkeys started to make history. It began with a series of experiments in which the monkeys, paralyzed in one hand, were separated into three distinct groups.

One group received good care, food and water, and a clean cage. But they received no rehabilitation, no therapy to get their hands moving again.

The second group received not only quality care, but also some basic therapy. They were taught how to move their arms, but were not given any exercises for individual finger movements or to perform any functional tasks, such as picking up a ball and throwing it, waving hello, or scratching their face. They didn't show any more improvement than the group who received no therapy at all. In other words, rudimentary therapy was as good as, well, nothing.

But the third group of monkeys was a different story. They received top-of-the-line "monkey rehab." They not only received the quality care of the first two groups, but they were also put to work: they were required to perform specific tasks that utilized individual fingers to pick and grab food pellets from small wells. And this group? *They did substantially better than the other two groups—and they had much more success in the return of the function of their paralyzed hands.*

This alone would show that the quality of rehabilitation is more important than the rehabilitation itself. But there's more:

When Dr. Nudo did sophisticated electrical stimulation studies on this last group of monkeys, they revealed something that was not seen in the other two groups. The area of the brain next to the damaged area was the place where shoulder movement was normally controlled. But now, in this third group of monkeys, this "shoulder movement locale" had increased in size—and had taken over the function of the hand.

In other words, the area of the brain that had been damaged (in this case the part that controlled hand movement) could no longer function and a different area of the brain took over the job.

The brain had literally rerouted its messages, transporting messengers away from the usual neurotransmitters and sending them down a different passageway—with ultimately the same result. In the same way a superhighway will change the course of the way a car will get from one town to another, the brain will change the way the message gets to where it needs to go.

But it gets there just the same.

Dr. Randolph J. Nudo and his monkeys had proved the rewiring of the brain, an exciting new aspect for stroke rehabilitation, offering new hope and new treatment options for those people who thought they might not be able to function at the same capacity as before.

Neural plasticity was born.

But First . . .

Although Dr. Nudo and his colleagues provided proof for the theory of neural plasticity, the idea of a flexible, resilient brain was formulated long before plastic was even a word in our dictionary.

In 1915, physician Shepherd Ivory Franz observed that many motor disabilities in people who had come to his hospital seemed to have occurred *after* the accident or stroke. In other words, the paralysis of a hand or a finger or a leg seemed to happen from a lack of use, not from an accident-induced inability. He called this phenomenon "uncared for paralysis" and, in 1917, he joined forces with another researcher, Dr. R. Ogden, and discovered that when the affected leg or arm was restrained (forced use therapy):

- Massaging the unrestrained affected limb showed absolutely no results . . .

■ . . . but forced use of the restrained leg or arm led to significant recovery.

Working with the theory of learned helplessness, Psychologist Martin Seligmann found that animals who failed to obtain positive feedback for their efforts eventually "gave up"—or learned helplessness. They just stopped trying.

Years later, in 1980, Dr. Edward Taub took these findings one step further and discovered that this learned nonuse was more destructive to successful rehabilitation than no rehabilitation at all. He began to formulate his theories of constraint therapy in which the paralyzed limb is forced into action.

How does this relate to neural plasticity?

Easy.

Let's go back to our new highway. In order to build that road, pour the concrete, and put up the railings, you need to know that cars will be using it. The highway has to be used. Otherwise, it will fall into disrepair from nonuse. Weeds will begin to peek out from the concrete; potholes will form; roadside stations will close up shop. The first route might have closed down from a traumatic accident or an "act of God," but the second route will have the same exact fate—if it's not used.

But if cars are forced to use that new highway, directed with arrows and signs and guards to go on this new road, they surely will. Eventually, they'll be humming along, the sun on the windshield, as if they'd always ridden on this road.

Brain plasticity and the new rehabilitation therapy have the exact same principles behind them:

By forcing rehabilitation patients to use the affected arm or leg, the brain is stimulated to reorganize its heady mass of synapses and neurotransmitters. It rewires a new route and literally takes charge: move that leg! But instead of, say, giving the command in French, it's now saying to do the job in English. Instead of taking Route 23, it's telling the message to take Highway 10.

The job gets done and rehabilitation does its work.

> "There are no hopeless situations; there are only men who have grown hopeless about them."
>
> —Claire Boothe Luce

The Gray Matter

Charlotte was not one for introspection. She had managed to live sixty-five years without major mishap. She'd raised two children and seen them graduate college and go on to successful careers. She had a good marriage that, if not always filled with fireworks, was strong and intimate. She had friends; she enjoyed her part-time job as a medical transcriber, and, although she never took fabulous vacations or traveled much away from home, she felt contented, happy, and fulfilled.

Of course, Charlotte's life wasn't always one long sunny day. She did have some health concerns that her doctor had kept telling her to keep in check. She had both diabetes and hypertension that she needed to take medication for—even though she walked at a brisk pace three times a week and tried to watch her diet.

Tried was the key word. Charlotte didn't always follow her doctor's advice—even though she did try. Some days, she'd forget to take her medicine. Other days, that dessert just seemed too tempting to forgo. After all, she felt great, she exercised on a regular basis, and she wasn't even overweight for her height and age.

Life was good for Charlotte and that was that.

Unfortunately, all that changed when she had her stroke. She'd been watching television with her husband; they were sharing some hot-air popcorn he'd just made and they were looking forward to seeing their favorite TV sitcom. One minute Charlotte was laughing at the characters on the TV screen; the next she was crumpled over in the chair.

Charlotte's contented life was officially over—or so she thought. The stroke changed everything for her. There were the weeks in the rehabilitation center, learning new skills and working very hard at retraining her body to go the way her mind wanted her to go. And, indeed, Charlotte made excellent progress. Her speech came back fairly rapidly. Her bladder and bowel were soon functioning normally. Her cognitive functions, her ability to remember and organize and think clearly, were fine. She learned to walk with a cane.

But Charlotte's arm was another story. Although her right side was perfectly fine, she could not move her arm on the left (hemiparesis). She worked and worked on her physical therapy exercises, first at an Encompass Health inpatient facility, then as an Encompass Health outpatient—to no avail. Charlotte was in despair, thinking that she'd never use her left hand again to do simple tasks like putting on makeup or donning a blouse. She became depressed—and displayed her pain and sadness by lashing out at her husband, her children, her friends. She lost interest in the things she once enjoyed. All she had left was her precious television and she watched it all her waking hours.

Charlotte's husband was extremely upset. He'd almost lost his wife to a stroke—and now he was afraid he'd lose her again. She wasn't herself; she was a stranger. An abusive, weepy stranger. But time has a way of healing things. Three months after Charlotte had her stroke, she suddenly noticed movement in her fingers. She could wiggle them slightly. It was slow going, but both Charlotte and her therapists were hopeful. She would get the movement in her left arm back!

Charlotte became herself again. Her depression lifted and she felt more optimistic about life. And then she hit the plateau. Weeks went by and there was no progress. None. Zero. All Charlotte could do was move her left arm slightly. More than just after the stroke, certainly, but not enough to do all of her daily routine.

But this story has a happy ending. Six months later her family insisted she try going to a stroke support group; it was something she had resisted in the past. She finally went. And surprise! She found that she actually looked forward to going to it. She became friends with many of the other members. They shared ideas and news items and emotions. At one evening's session, Charlotte heard about the Ness 200—a new way to retrain paralyzed limbs to move again by actually using electrical stimulation and forced use therapy so that the stroke survivor has to use the nonfunctioning limb.

Charlotte went back to her Encompass Health facility and talked to her occupational therapist about this therapy. After careful evaluation, she and the rest of Charlotte's rehabilitation team decided that Charlotte could be a good candidate for the Ness 200 and additional therapy. They decided to try it. Charlotte's unaffected right arm was put in a mitten, starting at sixteen hours each day. She couldn't use her unaffected arm for anything—and she was forced to use her weak left arm to brush her teeth, eat, dress, you name it. In addition she used the Ness 200 to help her perform functional tasks with her affected hand.

Within a few weeks, the plateau had disappeared. Charlotte began to use her left arm—without constraint. It wasn't a miracle; Charlotte couldn't suddenly rejoin her walking group at the mall. But she did find as the weeks went by that the paralysis of her left arm had improved significantly. She could now put on her own makeup. She could get dressed without her husband's help.

Charlotte no longer keeps her right arm in a mitten and she no longer has to "fight her brain" to use her left arm. Her left arm, although not functioning perfectly, moves when Charlotte wants it to. Her brain has marked a new highway to left arm movement and motor coordination; it was uncovered to do so by being forced to send messages to and from the affected arm.

She had done it. Charlotte felt great—and especially thankful that she lived in an exciting new world where the theories of neural plasticity and learned nonuse make movement a real and viable possibility for people who have had a stroke.

Plastic Molds

Like anything else in life, neural plasticity is not a perfect science. Many new technologies are being tried that include electrical stimulation and weight-supported treadmills. Numerous variables must be taken into account in order for this new rehabilitation to have the highest success rate:

Timing Is Everything

Think of a telephone cable network, a series of wires connecting one to the other, all interrelated and all connected to a main source. In many ways, the brain and its passageways are like a series of wires going this way and that way, all interconnected and coded by color. When you have a stroke, things stop. The connections between wires are immediately lost. Messages cannot get through. In order for the wires to reconnect—for instructions on, say, moving a hand, remembering a name, buttoning a blouse, to be understood and enacted—rehabilitation must start as soon as possible. When your phone goes out, it needs to be fixed yesterday. The same is true for your brain. The sooner rehab begins, the less time there is for the "dust to settle" and the connection to be lost forever.

A Wounded State

We've already seen how the location of a stroke is crucial to determining successful recovery after a stroke. But neural plasticity theories show that the location in the brain is not always as important as the location of the lesion in the neural network. In other words, if the stroke occurred on a crucial highway in the brain, even if it was, say, far from the king of executive function, the frontal cerebral cortex, the stroke would be serious. Messages would not be able to connect easily; network roads would not be able to connect.

And if that lesion were not only a roadblock on an important highway, but a big, traffic-stopping one, the success rate for recovery would be serious indeed.

The good news is that plasticity, by its very definition, means molding, growth, flexibility. Paths regenerate on their own; networks start up nearby; function returns on a different highway with proper rehabilitation as lesions heal.

Sci-Fi Thriller

Before the birds and the bees, there were sperm cells and egg cells. Those cells grew and developed into human beings, all of us with brains and hearts and lungs and limbs. Early on in this developmental process, we grow stem cells that, when turned on by certain growth factors, will turn into specific parts of our body. Scientists have actually learned how to harvest these stem cells and grow them, like tomatoes or roses, into brain cells, motor neurons, or spinal cord cells. When these new cells have been injected into the brains of animals in laboratory settings, the animals not only have survived, but some of the deficits caused by injury have healed. The nerve growth research has only just begun, but it holds much exciting promise for treating stroke and paralysis.

You Don't Eat These Sprouts

Think about your garden—or a garden you've seen on television. When you prune a bush or plant by cutting it back, the plant grows bigger, becomes more lush and healthier; it literally sprouts beautiful new growth. After a stroke, the wires in your brain, those axons and dendrites of a nerve cell, start sprouting new "stems," new growth to seek out new connections. This is called *collateral sprouting,* and this regeneration is an important element of neural plasticity. With good rehabilitation, those new stems can be trained to connect the correct way and traffic in the brain can hum along as it did before.

Learning New Things Every Day

When Dr. Nudo did his groundbreaking research with his monkeys, he discovered that it wasn't enough to retrain them to use their hands. As he said, "Changes in the motor cortex are driven by acquisition of new motor skills and not simply by motor use." In other words, it was not enough to have the monkeys tapping their fingers; he wanted them to learn to pick out food pellets from a well; he wanted them to learn to think, to figure out *how to* use their hands to get what they wanted.

The same principle applies in rehabilitation in humans. It isn't enough for you to use your weakened limb in physical therapy. You also have to do specific tasks, such as getting dressed or writing a note. By forcing your affected arm to work at different tasks, your brain becomes stimulated; the whole network surrounding the damaged area becomes active; highway branches (synapses and dendrites) sprout up; other areas of the brain pick up the functional slack.

Neural plasticity is an exciting new area of research—and this kind of rehabilitation has only just begun to see results. As with any new therapy, time will tell how precise it really is. Further studies need to be done to determine exactly when constraint therapy needs to begin, and how long it should be applied. Diagnostic tools must become as advanced as the research to know how much to do and when to begin.

But one thing is certain: there is hope and excitement and a new world waiting only a highway away. . . .

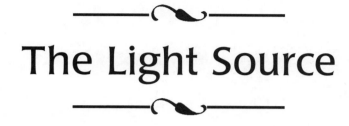

PART IV

The Light Source

CHAPTER 17

Family Business

> "I thank God every day he's alive. And I'm
> not complaining. It's just that, well, I didn't
> know it would be so tough. It feels as if my
> whole life is taking care of my husband. It's
> all I do."
>
> —*A retired schoolteacher and wife of a*
> *sixty-three-year-old stroke survivor*

Imagine this scenario.

It's the middle of the night. Your husband, sleeping next to you, cries out in his sleep. His body trembles. You jump out of bed, your face drained of color, and rush to the telephone. The ambulance takes him to the emergency room of your local hospital. You ride with him, your hand covering his.

The interminable waiting begins. One hour. Two. Sitting on those shiny plastic chairs, sipping coffee from a foam cup.

At last you get the news from the doctor. Your husband is alive. He has had a stroke. You hear words such as *left hemisphere, frontal lobe*. But they mean nothing. All you know is that he's alive, thank God.

Rehabilitation begins. Slowly but surely, your husband regains his ability to walk, with the aid of a cane. He regains his speech, his ability to read a book. He no longer is incontinent. Slowly but surely, he is beginning to function again.

Of course, there is the memory thing, the fact that he can't always remember your name. The therapist tells you that that might change in time. You wait and hope. Then there is the depression, those mood swings that your husband seems to have a lot. You don't know whether he'll be happy or sad or angry when you see him next.

Still, you wait and hope. You bury those other feelings, the anger, the despair, the frustration. They make you feel guilty.

But late at night, when no one can hear, you cry. You flash back on that other night, seemingly so long ago now, when your husband had his stroke. You remember it. You play it in your mind, and sometimes you don't know how you can go on.

He's home now, your husband. But he's not your husband. He's different. Everything is different: money, lifestyle, responsibility, everything. You're different, too. And you're tired, very tired.

Time passes. You've gotten used to the grab bars in the bathroom, the ramp to your front door. You've made peace with change. You can handle this. Sometimes.

Your husband smiles. He's alive. You are alive. Life is not perfect, not by any means, but it does have its rewards. You have grown. You have changed. And the bottom line is that the man you love still is alive. The nightmares have stopped.

This scenario is meant to be general, to only touch on some of the issues that come up when a loved one has a stroke: change, fear, doubt, exhaustion. A stroke brings these and more to the family sphere.

Taking Care of the Caretaker

Before you can take care of someone else, you have to take care of yourself. Doing so will give you a sense of well-being, a much-needed sense of control, and, most important of all, the strength to go on.

Some of the ways to "treat" yourself include:

- eating healthfully

- seeking professional help for your own emotional adjustment

- staying clear of alcohol and drug abuse

- taking time off to go to a movie or spend an evening with friends

- using private time wisely, for a soak in the tub, a massage, or even a luxurious middle-of-the-afternoon nap

- spending money on yourself, even if it's as small an item as a paperback book, a sports video, or a manicure

The distance and turmoil these issues bring in their wake can divide a family, just when support is needed the most. Without family support, rehabilitation will not be so successful. Studies have found that a stroke patient will not, without his family's help, make as much progress as he could. Conversely, dysfunctional families who are not supportive may hinder rehabilitation.

Furthermore, without family support, you, the caregiver, might be lost. As this illuminates, once the life-and-death question has been overcome, a whole host of other issues jumps in to take its place. Although not as crucial as life and death, they can create a great deal of stress, pain, and frustration. Economics, dependency needs, work questions, role reversal, unpredictable mood swings—all these can take a toll on the family—and on you. Without help, your emotional state can unravel. The family can disintegrate further, with each member feeling more and more alone.

Yes, a stroke changes the family structure. But change does not—and should not—mean disaster. With proper counseling, guidance, and understanding, not only can you provide the support that your loved one needs to make rehabilitation a success, but you can find the support that you so sorely need as well.

Family Ties

Before you can understand how a stroke affects the family, you have to first understand how the family unit is set up.

The family is the most basic, life-sustaining structure in society. The bond within a family is strong, and as anyone who has family problems knows, its ties are felt even if that bond is weakened. Because of this primal, almost instinctual, bond, there is an unconscious striving to maintain order, or balance, within the family. This "law and order" is maintained via an unspoken hierarchy, or pecking order, in which everyone has his role, everyone has his place. There might be one or two breadwinners, a nurturing caretaker, a teased younger sibling, even a scapegoat. As long as everybody knows his or her roles, peace is maintained and life in the family remains on an even keel.

But when the pecking order is disrupted, balance is lost. Tension and discord reign. Change, after all, threatens the continuation of the primal group, and it will be fought on both conscious and unconscious levels.

A stroke brings change. Its consequences can be highly disruptive and fraught with tension, especially when that stroke has occurred to the "leader of the pack," the person who has run the roost.

Stress enters the house, and until a new pecking order shifts into place, until a new balance is attained, the family players may feel anguish, anxiety, and pain in double doses: one dose for the

Family Ties

Not all family units are based on blood. In addition to the traditional nuclear family of husband, wife, and children, there are extended families, which include aunts and uncles, grandparents, even ex-spouses who have remained close. Alternative families also have strong bonds. These are single-parent homes, unmarried adults, and close friends.

Whatever the actual family makeup, the bond can be strong, close, and supportive. Family is family, regardless of the genes. When a stroke occurs, it is the family—nuclear, extended, or alternative—who can help most.

---

terrible tragedy that has befallen someone they love, and yet another for the frightening loss of family balance and identity.

In short, families need therapy and guidance as much as their loved one who has had a stroke. They, too, need counseling to understand and cope with their own feelings of grief and fear. They need to understand their anger and their subsequent guilt. They need to deal with the profound change that stroke has brought to everyone, in every arena of family life where balance once held center stage.

A Stroke Stress Analysis

Before we continue on to the problems that you and your family might face, look over these brief statements. If any of them sounds familiar, it's possible that the stress of your loved one's stroke is overwhelming at this time and additional family counseling could be in order to help you cope.

When a Stroke Occurs to a Husband or Wife

1. You cannot shake the feeling that a large part of yourself is lost forever.

2. Although your spouse has been home now for several months, you continue to turn down social engagements, becoming more and more isolated.

3. The responsibilities that you now bear alone are creating havoc on your emotions. You wake up repeatedly in the middle of the night with your heart pounding in fright.

4. Your economic state has grown worse as the months go by. You don't know where to turn.

5. You frequently dream of running away; you are beginning to feel hostility toward your spouse.

6. You haven't treated yourself well for months. Your appearance has deteriorated; your personal grooming has fallen by the wayside.

7. You are drinking and smoking more and more; you have lost your appetite. You have a feeling of not caring about anything.

8. You ignore your loved one when she asks for something.

9. You ignore the instructions of the rehabilitation team; you always make excuses about not seeing them.

10. You are lying to your coworkers, your friends, and your family about the progress that your loved one is making.

When a Stroke Occurs to a Parent

1. The added responsibility of an ailing parent may hit you at a very bad time: your own financial state, your marital woes, and your own children's problems may already be sources of stress.

2. You miss your parent the way he was before the stroke; you feel a terrible loss. The pain, instead of getting better over the past months, has grown worse.

3. You and your siblings are fighting too much among yourselves.

4. You feel that you shoulder more responsibility than anyone else in the family; you resent it, and your resentment is smoldering.

5. The old competitiveness that you and your brothers and sisters felt as children is coming back—in major fights and tears.

6. You aren't communicating with the rest of the family. No one is clear about what he or she wants and what he or she is doing. Everyone seems to be floundering.

7. Your feelings of anger and resentment toward your parent are starting to overpower you; they are influencing your care.

8. You spend less and less time with your parent. The guilt, the pain, the remorse—all of it simply hurts too much.

9. Your personal life is hurting; your health has deteriorated; you burst into tears at any given moment.

10. You escape in sleep—or alcohol or drugs.

Feeling or acting in any of these ways is not unusual if a loved one has had a stroke. But if this behavior continues for long periods of time with no relief, it could signal a depression, and you should call your physician. She is trained to recognize the warning signs of trouble. She can help you before your problems get worse and you no longer can cope.

Some other feelings that you may experience (as adapted from the Tampa General Rehabilitation Center's *Actions and Reactions: A Stroke Manual for Families*):

Feeling One: Panic

"Ohmigod, I can't handle this!"

Perhaps your heart beats faster because you don't know how far your health insurance will go. Perhaps you can't decide what to do, and you end up doing nothing. During the acute stages of your loved one's stroke, panic can set in, along with its terrifying loss of control and concentration.

Help. Focus on those aspects of your life that you can control. These can include small short-term personal goals, such as implementing an exercise or diet regime, or short-term job-related goals that can distract you from the problems at home. Reach out to friends, family, and the rehabilitation team. Accept the fact that you cannot change certain things; you can only do so much.

Feeling Two: Anxiety

"What if he needs me in the middle of the night and I can't hear him?"

Once your loved one has entered a rehabilitation facility, your initial panic might turn to anxiety. Suddenly, you begin to worry: Will he walk? Will he eat? Will he be able to get dressed? Perhaps you need to have the rehabilitation team explain every procedure several times before you find the confidence to try them out at home. Or perhaps your anxiety is irrational: you're terrified that you'll fail your loved one when he needs you most—again.

Help. Try relaxation techniques, such as deep breathing and meditation. Make sure that you take time off for yourself. Delegate responsibility as much as possible. Seek professional help.

Feeling Three: Denial That Leads to Overoptimism

"Oh, he'll be fine. He just needs to come home."

We already have seen denial at work, helping us avoid the very real, very terrible fact of our loved one's stroke. Unfortunately, this same denial can lead to a false sense of optimism, a delusion that all is well, that all will go back as before, that all will be over soon—by Christmas or by the spring at the very latest. But when the spring comes and things are *not* like they were, anger and depression can set in.

Help. Setting up realistic short-term and long-term goals can help. They help erase false beliefs head-on, while, at the same time, they bolster motivation as, for example, your loved one moves an arm, buttons a shirt, or makes a sandwich. Listen to what the rehabilitation team is telling you.

Feeling Four: Irritability and Anger

"It's all the rehabilitation team's fault!"

Once you are forced to face your denial and its subsequent disappointment, you may replace it with anger. Suddenly, you are furious with the entire situation—and everyone involved, from the physician on down. Perhaps you blame the staff for your loved one's slow progress. Perhaps you are angry at your loved one for "deserting" you. Perhaps you are angry at him for his incontinence; he is embarrassing you.

On the other hand, your anger might be more of a slow boil rather than an outburst, an irritating gnawing that won't go away.

The Seven Deadly Stroke Impacts on Family Life

1. Physical. The family's energy is completely focused on the stroke victim. Role reversal is taking place.

2. Psychological. A complex myriad of feelings, from guilt to depression, are sifting through each member of the family.

3. Emotional. The emotions within the family can change from day to day, from hour to hour, from ambivalence to anger, from frustration to anxiety.

4. Social. The family's role in the community begins to change. Normal social patterns are interrupted or ceased. Isolation can set in as one's friends return to their normal lives.

5. Economic. Financial stresses are obvious within the family. These can include loss of income, health-insurance snafus, and increased costs of uncovered expenses, such as home equipment, parking at the hospital, and more.

6. Spiritual. Many families turn to God in difficult times such as these. They might question their beliefs.

7. Sexual. Sex can change after stroke, affecting every other aspect of your family's life—and its sense of loss.

Adapted from Kozy, M. C. and Tarvin, G. A., "Working with Families," in *Clinical Management of Right Hemisphere Dysfunction* by M. S. Burns, A. S. Halper, and S. I. Mogil, eds., p. 98, with permission of Aspen Publishers, Inc., © 1985.

This can result in impatience, ungrounded complaining, and feelings of frustration.

Help. Realize that the anger you feel is a common reaction. Rational or irrational, it still is a feeling that many people experience. As you become aware of your anger, try to control it, especially when it is directed at the wrong person. Evaluate what it is that you are really upset about. Is it your loss of control? The dramatic changes in your life? Seek out professional help if the anger persists.

Setting Goals

Whether short-term or long-term, goals must be realistic. Talk to the members of the rehabilitation team to help set appropriate goals for you and your loved one. They should fall into four groups.

1. Physical. These goals should involve the basics—mobility, speech, and the simple activities of daily living.

2. Recreational. You'll need to determine whether your loved one can return to his prior leisure activities. Will he need to adapt the way he gardened on Sunday afternoons? Will he be able to drive? What about his golf game?

3. Family. A stroke survivor should participate in family functions as much as possible. A goal here can include, for example, preparing a meal or washing the dishes. These goals can be as simple as helping to decide what presents to send for birthdays and holidays.

4. Personal. Everyone should strive for their personal best, and a person who has had a stroke is no exception. Perhaps your loved one will want to drive again someday; his short-term realistic goal might be passing the driving evaluation at his facility. Perhaps he would like to write a letter; his short-term realistic goal can be putting down a few sentences on paper. Although limitations must be addressed, compromise is always possible. Remember: realistic goals bolster self-esteem.

Feeling Five: Frustration

"I can't stand one more thing going wrong!"

Anger and frustration are partners in a world where stress is constant and change has abruptly instigated a new way of life. Because stroke recovery can take a long time, patience can wear thin. Because functional recovery sometimes can go only so far, frustration can overwhelm you. And, as with anything in life, the outside world can add its own frustration triggers: an insurance company that won't pay for rehabilitation services, a lack of support in your community, a plateau in rehabilitation progress.

Help. Identify individual problems and work with your rehabilitation team to solve them—one at a time. The team will also help provide feedback and understanding: you are not alone. And, as you find solutions with their help, your stress will decrease.

Feeling Six: Fatigue

"I'm utterly, completely exhausted from the experience."

Of course, you're tired. Not only do you have the emotional stress that the stroke has created, but you have very real physical stress as well: making countless trips to the doctor; setting up a safe environment in your house; planning an outpatient routine for your loved one at home, including interviewing and hiring housekeepers; helping your loved one perform the activities of daily living, which now take twice as long; not to mention your loved one's *own* very real and equally overwhelming physical and emotional fatigue.

Indeed, there is so much to do, so much to worry about, that you might push yourself too far. Fatigue can turn into complete overexhaustion, which won't do anyone any good.

Help. Relax! Take time out for yourself. Prioritize. Only do those things that absolutely need to be done first. Delegate responsibilities. You might not believe it, but most people want to help. When people ask what they can do, tell them. Give them a specific task, such as driving your loved one to his therapist.

Feeling Seven: Hopelessness and Helplessness

"What's the use? Nothing's going to change."

Sometimes it occurs when the cycle of denial and overoptimism is lifted, when you realize that some of the disabilities your loved one now has will not resolve. Sometimes it occurs further on in the rehabilitation process, when progress slows down, when improvement is negligible. But whenever depression does occur, the feeling of hopelessness or helplessness can be debilitating—and you may need professional help.

Help. Trite but true: sometimes keeping busy is the best medicine. As difficult as it can seem at times, keeping up your daily routines will help. Doing the shopping, the laundry, the cleaning, and the cooking are all mundane, yes, but they help provide structure and connect you to the world. Try to reestablish the parts of your life that existed before the stroke: your bridge game, your gardening club, your classes.

Other suggestions: look at what you want for your loved one. Are you expecting too much? Are you being unrealistic? Modify your goals and your expectations. Accept the fact that *function* is a relative term: things may be different, but they can still have their own set of joys and triumphs. If, despite your best efforts, your feelings of despondency continue and you cannot see hope anywhere along the way, seek out professional help. Your rehabilitation team manager can offer you some recommendations.

Feeling Eight: Guilt

"How can I be so angry at him? It's not fair. I'm a horrible person."

Guilt thrives on trauma and stress. And a loved one's stroke fits the bill perfectly: it's all my fault. If I hadn't had a fight with my husband that day, none of this would have happened. Or later on in the process: I'm not doing enough. If I were a better, happier, more accomplished, smarter, and really, really good person, my wife would be better by now.

Guilt is always waiting in the wings. An angry thought directed at your loved one can easily turn to guilt: how can I be angry at my husband? He's ill. I love him. He's trying so hard.

Guilt doesn't need to be self-imposed. People around you may unwittingly supply guilt's fuel, offering suggestions that you are "plain foolish not to take" and judging the way that you're handling things. Carefully weigh the advice of friends and family. Remember, they are not you, and they are not in your situation.

Help. Guilt can be a common reaction to a loved one's stroke. Accept it, but don't let it consume you. Quickly identify its source and seek help from your rehabilitation counselor as soon as you recognize it for what it is. Seek out friends or stroke groups who offer support, not judgments. Talking to someone who has been where you are right now can make all the difference in the world.

Feeling Nine: Ambivalence

"I don't know how I feel anymore. I can't make a decision about anything."

In short, ambivalence is experienced when what you feel you should do conflicts with what you want to do. It's easy to see where this can fit into life with a loved one who has had a stroke. You feel that you should be more patient in helping your husband dress, but you don't feel like doing it anymore. You know that you still should care for your wife, but, sometimes, you just don't know if love really is there anymore. With all this ambivalence floating around, it's no wonder that suddenly you feel trapped and unable to make a decision about anything!

Help. This is a tough one to do on your own. Take advantage of the expert counselors available at your rehabilitation facility. To help make the best choices, use people you respect and trust as sounding boards. Rather than always asking yourself "What if?" imagine the worst possible scenario. Seeing and visualizing it can take away the fear. You've turned the light on the "monsters" and they aren't as bad as you had thought. Ultimately, whatever decision you make, you've faced the worst in your mind's eye and you can handle it.

Stroke Support

A stroke club or support group's main goal is to provide just that: support—plus encouragement, compassion, and friendship to all the members of a stroke survivor's family. Meetings are usually held once a month.

Although they are similar in their goals, there is a difference. Stroke clubs are organized and designed by stroke survivors and their families. Support groups, on the other hand, usually are run by the rehabilitation hospitals themselves and supervised by a health care professional.

A support group might be more beneficial during the rehabilitation process, when thoughts and feelings are most confusing. Later, when you and your loved one have settled back in at home, a more socially oriented, community-minded stroke club might be the best choice.

One final note: remember that you are not alone. The feelings you are experiencing might be strong, but they are not inappropriate. They are quite normal for your situation. You are being forced to adjust to a fundamental change in your family life and in your own personal way of viewing the world. This may not come easy, but many have successfully negotiated this path.

Family Unity

A rehabilitation team is not only there for the person who has had a stroke. It is also an invaluable resource for the family. It's a true give-and-take. Families help a team individualize their patient's rehabilitation program, providing feedback and insight into who the person was before the stroke. The rehabilitation team, in turn, is there for the family. Here's what families need and what they can expect from their rehabilitation team:

1. **Encouragement to ask questions—and more questions.**
    No matter how simple the questions might sound to you, it's
    important you don't feel intimidated to ask away.

2. **Information, information, information**—as much infor-
    mation as you could ever need or want. The more you know,
    the more you learn, the better able you will be to cope and
    help your loved one, too.

3. **Extra training for the primary caregiver,** the key person
    who provides assistance at home. Family training is critical
    for a smooth transition home. The rehabilitation team will
    teach you to properly transfer or assist your loved one. They
    will also accompany you on "training trips" back home—
    and provide invaluable feedback on your return; this will
    help you improve not only your caregiving skills, but your
    confidence levels as well.

4. **A social worker or a case manager assigned to your
    family, a person who will specifically work with all of
    you—individually and together.** This person will help you
    through the maze of insurance, home health agencies, medi-
    cal equipment companies, and more.

5. **Resource material and support groups.** The rehabilitation
    team is trained to know what's available in your community
    and when. They will be able to assist you in finding educa-
    tional materials such as this book, transportation services,
    meal services, vocational referral services, community get-
    togethers, stroke clubs, and more.

6. **Sensitivity to know where each family member is in the
    grieving process—and knowing when to try to move for-
    ward as well as when not to push.** One family member

might still be in shock. A different family member might be ready to forge ahead. A team will work with you wherever you are.

This, then, in brief, is a general look at you—the family who must cope with and accept a loved one's stroke. But before we close, we'd like to offer some specifics, some actual situations within the family that may arise—and some information on how best to handle them. They are coming up in Chapter 18.

Family Problems . . . and Solutions

"Simple things. Like setting up the bathroom
and the kitchen for my dad to get around
and help. It made life easier for all of us."
—*Daughter of a sixty-two-year-old landscaper*
who had a stroke

Our journey is almost at an end. Throughout these pages, we have tried to touch on the most important issues involved in stroke. We have tried to address its physical manifestations, what stroke is, and how it works. We have discussed diagnosis, pharmacological treatments, risk factors, and the entire rehabilitation spectrum—from physical therapy and activities of daily living to the impact of stroke on family life. Before we close, we'd like to examine some of the more common problems that have cropped up at our rehabilitation facilities, the questions, and the answers that have surfaced among the families whose lives have been touched by stroke.

Here are some of these family matters.

Family Matters One

"My husband had been incontinent for a long time. Now that he's home from the rehabilitation hospital, he still has accidents now and then. How do I cope with this?"

As we saw in Chapter 14, incontinence is a common problem in stroke survivors. Most patients do regain the ability to void, but unfortunately, some people remain on automatic. Their brains cannot coordinate the information that they need to store urine in their bladder or wait once they feel an urge. First, be certain the situation has been adequately evaluated; make sure your husband is free of infection. Has a urologist reviewed his case? A post void residual (PVR) should be checked to see if the bladder completely empties after he has urinated. If there is a problem, there is help available. Medications can aid the ability to empty or store urine. Offering a urinal or the opportunity to go to the bathroom every two hours while awake and limiting intake of fluids after 6:00 at night can make a world of difference.

The most important thing to remember is that incontinence can try both your patience and the patience of your loved one. Most of our sense of self-esteem is related to our ability to perform our own activities of daily living. Obviously, bladder and bowel function are closely tied to that self-esteem. Be patient. And don't be embarrassed to seek help.

Family Matters Two

"My wife had a stroke two years ago. Ever since then, she's been erratic, her moods swinging from elation to tears. How do I handle this?"

Emotional highs and lows can be very unsettling. A change in personality can threaten the most peaceful family's balance. But when that change *keeps* happening, day by day, it does more than threaten; it can completely disrupt a family.

It's important to realize that these emotional swings do not mean that your loved one feels more than she used to feel. Rather, it means that the parts of her brain that keep her emotions in check have been damaged.

Perhaps when she sees a family member or a friend, she responds by immediately crying. Or perhaps she'll laugh for no reason at all. Whatever the situation, it can be extremely unsettling for a family that is already trying to keep its own emotions in check. Unfortunately, simple reassurances don't always work. Your loved one may not understand; she can't help herself. She might react by crying or laughing even more, which will, in turn, make communication even more difficult.

Instead of words, try putting your arm on your wife's shoulder when she starts to cry. Distracting her by changing the topic frequently brings outbursts to a stop. Or simply ignore them. They will pass. Medication sometimes reduces the severity of this emotional lability—talk to your doctor.

Family Matters Three

"My rehabilitation case manager mentioned making our home environment more handicap-accessible. But I'm not sure what this means and how I can make my father comfortable and independent without it costing a fortune."

An accessible environment is one that is structurally sound, safe, and barrier-free for a stroke survivor who might have trouble walking, who is confined to a wheelchair, or who is weak or paralyzed on one side of his body. A therapist from the rehabilitation facility may make a house call to determine what needs to be done; she can also offer suggestions based on your description of your home. These include the following:

- Doorways should be at least 32 inches wide to allow wheelchair access. If this a problem in your home, molding, hinges, and the doors themselves can be removed.

- Keep electrical cords and telephone wires tucked away in corners so that they can't be tripped over.

- Remove all throw rugs. They are the number-one cause of falls among the elderly.

- Keep nightlights on in all rooms so that you and your loved one can move around more easily in the dark.

- Before buying any equipment, check with your case manager or therapist. Make sure that the devices you want to purchase are necessary. Shop around for the best price.

- A ramp might be necessary if you have steps leading up to your front and back doors. The ramp should be one foot in length for every one inch in vertical rise.

- Telephones should be easily reached; emergency telephone numbers should be written in large print and placed at each extension.

- Counter heights in the kitchen might need to be adjusted or additional space built. Kitchen appliances, the washer and dryer, microwave ovens—these, too, will need to be placed at an accessible level.

- Keep kitchen utensils, plates, silverware, and glasses in easy reach. Condiments and canned foods should be on the lowest shelf of cabinets that should be at arm height.

- The bathroom might need modification to ease movement between toilet, bath, and wheelchair. Some of the equipment might include a shower chair, grab bars, a handheld shower, and safety rails. Soap on a rope is convenient for showers.

■ If possible, use a downstairs room for the stroke survivor's bedroom. Keep a bell or buzzer nearby on the night table. Lifeline call systems that are worn around the neck for contacting 911 can usually be obtained through your local hospital.

■ Bed height and width will need to be checked. Transferring to and from the bed to the wheelchair must be comfortably and easily performed.

■ Rearrange furniture so that a wheelchair can easily maneuver around chairs, sofas, and tables. Remove deep pile carpeting.

Family Matters Four

"My husband is impatient. He wants to get back into the car and start driving again. How do I know if this is safe or not?"

Medical clearance to drive is required after a person has had a stroke. Physical disabilities, visual and perceptual deficits, or poor judgment can all impair the ability to drive. Driver evaluation is based on a two-step performance:

Step One: The Predriving Test. Here, physical skills such as coordination, sensation, strength, and reaction time are checked. Vision is tested for both day and night. Perceptual and cognitive abilities are evaluated via interviews and standardized testing.

Step Two: Behind-the-Wheel Exam. This is a typical driver's education test. Your loved one sits behind the wheel; a driving instructor sits on the passenger side of the car. The automobile itself may have dual controls; it is modified to allow for physical impairments, such as braking and steering devices. The test may take place during daylight or at night.

Family Matters Five

"My wife has been home from the hospital for months now, but she continues to be tired all the time. She has no strength. What can I do?"

Fatigue is a common complaint after stroke, especially if the patient is older, less active, and overweight before the onset of the stroke. Furthermore, the various exercises and routines that she must do to get her cognitive and perceptual skills back can be mentally exhausting. Combined, they can create overwhelming fatigue—in everyone.

As the caregiver, you have to watch your impatience level. Fatigue is real; your wife is not faking it to get attention. Plan the day with rest periods and naps. Pick activities that don't cause more fatigue; don't pack your days with errands and shopping with no relief from crowds. Have people over to the house, but make sure they understand that they'll be "ordered out" before dinner; tell your guests beforehand that they'll need to leave at a specified time.

As seen in Chapter 10, your doctor may prescribe medicine to help alleviate the fatigue and help her stay more alert during the day.

Family Matters Six

"It doesn't matter what I cook or what restaurant we'll go to. My husband just won't eat. He won't eat. Help!"

Chances are, your husband is not faking it; he has lost his appetite. He's just not hungry. The damage done in the brain can cause this decrease in appetite, especially in right-hemisphere strokes. In fact, during the early stages of stroke rehabilitation, his therapists most likely spent a great deal of time getting him to swallow, to eat again, and to get the nourishment that he needed.

A loss of appetite also can have a psychological root. Your husband might be embarrassed by the way that he now eats, the way he handles a knife or fork, or the way that he chews and swallows. Depression, too, can frequently result in weight loss and a loss of interest in food.

To rule out other conditions, make sure your doctor has checked for stomach problems. Ask him about medicines that can stimulate the appetite, such as Megace® or Periactin®. If your husband seems to be depressed (see Chapter 15), make sure he gets the professional help he needs.

Family Matters Seven

"My mother still has a problem with her memory. She seems disoriented. I feel helpless when I visit her. It breaks my heart."

Although memory loss can be common after multiple strokes, it doesn't make it any less difficult to bear. Sometimes, it clears up spontaneously; sometimes, lives must adjust. Some tips to deal with memory loss include the following:

- A relaxed and calm environment can help. Too much stimulation will only confuse your mother and she won't be able to concentrate on the compensatory strategies that she's already learned for her memory loss.

- Speak clearly as you enter the room. Smile, say hello, and talk slowly. Repeat yourself, if necessary, in the same tones. Gestures can frequently communicate much of your message.

- Use tags on your mother's belongings to help her remember what they are. Chair, shampoo, brush—all can have their labels.

- Keep dates, times, and important occasions clear in your mother's mind with large calendars, a large-faced clock, and a memory book.

- Avoid correcting your mother's mistakes too much. Use questions that can be easily answered with yes or no to help her feel successful—and keep her motivation up.

- Remember: this is your parent, not your child. Do not speak down to her. She is still the same compassionate and intelligent woman who helped raise you.

Family Matters Eight

"I want my brother to help with the chores now that he's home. I feel it will do him a great deal of good, with the added plus that it will help me. But how do I get him to help?"

Asking your loved one to participate in daily chores will help immeasurably in the rehabilitation process. Not only does this reinforce independence and a sense of self-control, but it prevents him from feeling like a burden. Some suggestions follow:

- Use an electric can opener in the kitchen. If you put a piece of foam under the can, it can be used with one hand.

- Use a lapboard as a cutting board; it can be balanced on the arms of a wheelchair.

- Keep mixing bowls from slipping by using a nonslip rubberized mat.

- Keep premeasured amounts of laundry detergent and softeners within easy reach. Keep the washer and dryer level with the wheelchair. Use front-opening machines and rolling laundry carts.

- Ask your loved one to pick out produce and foods at the deli, fish, and meat counters. They usually are at shoulder level and are staffed with people who slice and cut what you order.

Family Matters Nine

"My husband is driving me crazy. He's angry all the time, irritable. Like he's a ten-year-old boy having a tantrum. What can I do?"

As we have seen, emotional swings are difficult to take, especially when they involve someone you love. Even though you know it's the stroke talking, not the man you fell in love with and married, it still hurts, particularly because this "stranger" is a new person, a different person. Perhaps your loved one throws things at the slightest frustration. Perhaps he screams obscenities at you. Perhaps he screams until he gets what he wants.

The best way to handle these temper outbursts is with a calm attitude. Use a calm voice, a calm action. Gently steer your loved one away from his focus of agitation. Distract him with something else, perhaps television or a magazine. Your physician can also prescribe medications to help calm these storms. Above all, do not take it personally. Your husband can't help himself.

Family Matters Ten

"My father is depressed. It's understandable, but I don't know how to get him out of it. All he wants to do is withdraw. He doesn't want to talk to anyone. Worse, he has no motivation to do anything."

Withdrawal, lack of motivation, depression—these all are signs of trouble, and they can all be common in poststroke patients. As we have seen in earlier sections, depression is not something you should deal with on your own. You need to discuss the problem with a physician. Some strategies that might help include:

- Go to a stroke club meeting with your father.

- Draw him out by planning activities that he likes to do. Maybe he likes to garden or listen to opera. Whatever—as long as it is not too taxing.

- Take him out on day trips even when he just passively sits there and says nothing. The distraction will be beneficial.

- Add structure to his day by making a schedule and following it.

- Most important of all: ask your doctor to prescribe an antidepressant medication. The newer drugs can lead to remarkable changes within two weeks to a month.

Family Matters Eleven

"My husband is incredible. All he can think about is me, me, me. 'How could my wife just leave me tonight and go play bridge?' 'Who cares what they want for dinner tonight? I'm the one who's sick!' He just won't let up!"

It's a fact. Many people become self-centered after a stroke. They revert back to their childhood, to the days when the world really did revolve around their every action. They see everything from only their own perspective and their own needs. Unfortunately, as an adult, this behavior is not endearing or cute, especially to a family whose emotions have already been taxed to the limit. The best antidote is other people; stroke clubs and support groups are particularly good for helping stroke survivors put things into perspective. When people ask what they can do, tell them to visit, take your husband out to lunch, or anything else that can relieve you for a well-deserved break. Maintain your own regular schedule to avoid "caregiver burnout."

Family Matters Twelve

"My wife is terrified all the time. I don't even know half the time what she's afraid of. She clings to me constantly."

As you already know by now, a stroke changes many old habits. Some of these changes occur because of physical reasons, because of damage done to the brain. But other changes have a psychological basis. Perhaps your wife is uncomfortable renewing old friendships; she might not be ready to make new friends. Right now, all she knows is that she feels comfortable with you and she clings to that.

This social dependency may also be connected to her fears, fear that she will have another stroke, fear that you no longer find her attractive, fear that she will no longer be included in your life.

Added to this mix is the age factor, the normal fears that we all have as we grow older. Will I have the same energy? What if I'm dependent on my children? What if I get sick and can't work? These fears are compounded when a stroke occurs; it is a nightmare coming true.

The best advice is two words: *consistency* and *encouragement*. Reassure your wife that you still love who she is by complimenting her abilities and skills whenever you can. Find things she can be successful doing, such as arranging flowers, cooking, or organizing the family room, and suggest she do them. Be patient and control your temper as much as possible. Always use praise when the situation calls for it. Join a stroke club or support group with your wife. Meeting other people with the same fears will go far in helping her—and you—through this difficult time. Try to be optimistic; see the cup as half-full and focus on her abilities, not on her disabilities. Remember, as we saw in Chapter 15, optimism can be learned.

Family Matters Thirteen

"I'm confused with the different terms that are thrown around whenever anyone brings up rehabilitation. What's the difference between an *impairment,* a *disability,* and a *handicap*—and how do they influence my finances?"

On a personal level, labels mean nothing. But, from a legal standpoint, they can make a big difference. *Impairment* implies the loss of normal functions, such as a paralyzed arm or leg. A *disability* is an inability to perform a specific activity in what we consider a "normal" way; a person's paralyzed arm, for example, interferes with his ability to tie a shoe or open a jar. A *handicap* is a descriptive word used for both impairments and disabilities that implies a societal disadvantage. Perhaps, because of your disability, you can no longer compete for the same job as before. Special drivers' licenses, laws protecting the rights of the differently abled, and handicap access laws are all designed to protect those with disabilities.

The good news is that whether your loved one's symptoms are labeled as an impairment, a disability, or a handicap, financial support can be found. Case managers are quite knowledgeable in helping you find what is available.

Family Matters Fourteen

"It's not even that I don't want to make love anymore. It's not that. I really believe that I want to go my separate way. How can I tell him that I want a divorce after all he's been through . . . all we've been through . . . with his stroke?"

Sometimes it happens. All the advice, the therapies, and the optimistic attitudes cannot always rebuild a relationship. If your marriage is hurting, chances are that the stroke is not the primary problem. Of course, the stroke can change the person you once loved—which can leave you wondering if you are now married to a stranger. But, most likely, your severed ties were a long time in coming, way before the stroke occurred—which can make you resent the role of caregiver you are now thrust into even more.

If you feel that divorce is inevitable, we strongly suggest that you speak to your physician or psychologist about it. She might want you to wait until your loved one is stronger; legally, a stroke survivor might not be currently competent to make independent decisions. Your doctor will also be able to give you some names of therapists for you to consult; she will help better prepare you and your loved one, both on a practical level and on an emotional level.

Family Matters Fifteen

"I know that stroke is common in the elderly, but what about young people? Do children get strokes, too?"

Five percent of the strokes that occur in America affect persons younger than forty-five. Some of them are as young as two years old.

The diseases and conditions that have been associated with the risk of stroke in younger people include:

- congenital heart conditions

- mitral valve prolapse

- infectious endocarditis

- arrhythmic heart conditions such as atrial fibrillation

- sickle-cell anemia

- rheumatic fever

- leukemia

- drug abuse, including cocaine and intravenous drugs

There also are some cases where strokes simply occur, a twist of fate where no disease, no congenital condition, is present. For these young people, the prognosis for a healthy, long life is excellent once rehabilitation is completed.

Family Matters Sixteen

"When friends ask me what they can do, I'm at a loss. I want everything and then some, but I don't want to be a burden."

Although we need the support of family and friends when the stroke occurs, it is not in the acute care hospital that their help is needed most. It is later, when your loved one returns home from the rehabilitation facility. It is then, when you might feel overwhelmed and alone, that you need the support of your friends. Ask them to come over and visit. Ask them to take your loved one to a restaurant—and give you some much-needed downtime. Ask them to take over some of the responsibility while you go out and get your hair cut or buy a new shirt or dress. We all need these treats and the time to enjoy them. So when friends call while your loved one is in the hospital and ask what they can do, say, "Nothing right now, but when she comes home, I could sure use your help."

Family Matters Seventeen

"What about dental care?"

Taking care of one's teeth is always important—but a stroke can make it a more difficult task. Memory loss, difficulty swallowing and chewing, lack of sensation, limited range of arm motion—all these can create problems in someone who has had a stroke. The best solution is the same as with all of us: dental visits two or three times a year. Some special considerations include these:

- Make sure the dentist's office is accessible.

- Ask the dentist to write down any instructions.

- If memory loss is a problem, have your loved one keep a daily log that he can check off when he brushes and flosses his teeth.

- Investigate one-handed aids, such as a one-handed dental flosser, electric toothbrushes, and jet-air Water Piks.

Family Matters Eighteen

"What about fun? It seems like such a challenge."

Entertainment is in the eye of the receiver. And laughter can come in unexpected places. Some suggestions follow:

- Keep radio, books, magazines, and television controls within easy reach. Remote controls now come with oversize buttons for easy visibility and use.

- Attach Post-It Notes with telephone numbers of friends next to the telephone; speed dialing and speaker telephones are especially helpful. This way your loved one can call and chat with a friend without asking you for help.

- Encourage your loved one to join a health club or a local YMCA that has a swimming pool.

- Play games! Some that come to mind are Scrabble, Nintendo, Myst, chess, checkers, bridge, Yahtzee, Pictionary, Trivial Pursuit—in short, any game that can help improve spatial perception, memory, problem-solving skills, and organizational ability.

- Go away—often. Vacations and a change of scenery are as important as ever. But always check to make sure that your planned destination is accessible. Always call ahead and ask:

  Is there handicapped-accessible parking?

  Is there a handicapped-accessible hotel room?

  What does your airline provide for their passengers with disabilities?

  Are there building ramps? How wide are the doorways?

  Are there handicapped-accessible bathroom facilities?

  Are there carpets? How heavy is the pile?

There are travel organizations that provide information for all people with disabilities, including stroke survivors. You can reach Flying Wheels by telephone at (877) 451-5006, by fax at (507) 451-1685, or via their website: www.flyingwheelstravel.com. Mobility International helps provide overseas jobs for people in wheelchairs; they can be reached by phone at (541) 343-1284, by fax at (541) 343-6812, via their e-mail address at info@miusa.org, or by visiting their website: www.miusa.org.

These are just a few of the family matters that can crop up during your loved one's recovery. Check the Appendix in the back of the book for other resources. And, as always, ask your case manager or physician any and all questions that come to mind. They are there to help you.

Beyond Stroke

If there is one lesson to be learned from this book, one statement to bring home, it is that, yes, the moment your loved one felt the first signs of a stroke, a profound change occurred.

But is that change an impossible one to deal with?

No.

A debilitating change that prevents you from moving forward?

No.

Life is not always fair.

But as long as there is breath, as long as there is even the memory of the person you love in the face that sleeps in the hospital bed, as long as there is the occasional smile, the gesture that you remember from holidays long past, from Sunday afternoons, from times well shared—as long as there are these, there is hope.

There is life.

You and your loved one should not give up as long as there is that hope. Yes, you might need help. But life has not ended. It does not have to become impossible. It has just changed.

We hope that this book has given you a solid base in stroke education. We hope that you now understand how your loved one's stroke began—and why. We hope that you now understand the many diagnostic tests that various physicians and health care professionals perform in the hospital.

We hope, too, that you have learned to ask the right questions about rehabilitation. We hope that you have learned that the rehabilitation team is there for you—and that you needn't be ashamed, embarrassed, or afraid to ask them anything at all.

But before we close, we would like to add one more word to your stroke vocabulary: *dignity.*

Yes, your loved one is different after a stroke. But it does not erase all that you have been or all you will be together. Nor should it weaken the bonds that tie a family together. Treat each other with the same dignity you would want offered to you.

It will not only help the rehabilitation process, but, we suspect, it might even add something to your life, too.

Useful Addresses for Education and Support

American Heart Association
National Center
7272 Greenville Avenue
Dallas, TX 75231
(214) 373-6300
(800) 373-AHA-USA1 (242-8721)
www.americanheart.org

American Occupational Therapy Association
4720 Montgomery Lane
P.O. Box 31220
Bethesda, MD 20824-1220
(301) 652-2682
www.aota.org

American Physical Therapy Association
1111 North Fairfax Street
Alexandria, VA 22314
(800) 999-2782
www.apta.org

American Speech-Language-Hearing Association
2200 Research Boulevard
Rockville, MD 20850
(800) 638-8255
(301) 296-5700 (Voice or TTY)
www.asha.org

American Stroke Association
7272 Greenville Avenue
Dallas, TX 75231
1 (888) 4-STROKE
www.strokeassociation.org

Association of Rehabilitation Nurses
4700 West Lake Avenue
Glenview, IL 60025-1485
(800) 229-7530
www.rehabnurse.org

Brain Injury Association of America
1608 Spring Hill Road
Vienna, VA 22182
(800) 444-6443 (family help)
(703) 761-0750 (business office)
www.biausa.org

Encompass Health
9001 Liberty Parkway
Birmingham, AL 35242
(800) 765-4772
www.encompasshealth.com

Encompass Health Rehabilitation Hospital of San Antonio
9119 Cinnamon Hill
San Antonio, TX 78240
(210) 691-0737

The Joint Commission
One Renaissance Boulevard
Oakbrook Terrace, IL 60181
(630) 792-5000
(630) 792-5800
www.jointcommission.org

Joseph P. Kennedy Jr. Foundation
1133 19th Street NW, 12th Floor
Washington, DC 20036-3604
(202) 393-1250
www.jpkf.org

Learning Disabilities Association of America
4156 Library Road
Pittsburgh, PA 15234
(888) 300-6710
(412) 341-1515
www.ldaamerica.org

The Moody Foundation
2302 Post Office Street, Suite 704
Galveston, TX 77550
(409) 797-1500
www.moodyf.org

National Aphasia Association
350 Seventh Avenue, Suite 902
New York, NY 10001
(800) 922-4622
www.aphasia.org

National Stroke Association
9707 East Easter Lane
Centennial, CO 80112
(800) 787-6537
www.stroke.org

TASH (association for persons with disabilities and families)
1025 Vermont Avenue NW, Suite 300
Washington, DC 20005
(202) 540-9020
www.tash.org

Medical Devices and Assistive Equipment

Sammons Preston
1000 Remington Boulevard, Suite 210
Bolingbrook, IL 60440-5117
(800) 475-5036
(800) 547-4333 (fax)
www.sammonspreston.com

Superintendent of Documents
P.O. Box 371954
Pittsburgh, PA 15250-7954
(866) 512-1800
(202) 512-1800
http://bookstore.gpo.gov

Documents available on disability law, health insurance, and the physically challenged

Glossary

Abduction. Movement of the arm or hip sideways away from the body.

Abstract concept. A concept that is disassociated from any specific instance and may therefore be difficult to understand. Patients with cognitive deficits usually have difficulty with abstract concepts. Thus, explanations should focus on concrete concepts utilizing immediate experience of actual things or events.

Adduction. Movement of arm or leg sideways toward the body.

ADLs (activities of daily living). Tasks performed every day in order for a person to care for himself. These include bathing, grooming, dressing, feeding, toileting, communication, light meal preparations, homemaking, as well as prevocational/vocational skills.

Affect. The emotional reactions associated with an experience.

AFO. Ankle-foot orthosis; a short leg brace.

Agitation. Internal confusion that may result in defensive behavior, excessive restlessness, and increased mental and physical activity, including some tremors.

Alertness. Responsiveness to inputs from the environment.

Alexia. Inability to understand written language.

Amnesia. Lack of memory about events occurring during a particular period of time.

Aneurysm. Localized abnormal dilation of a blood vessel, usually an artery, due to a congenital defect or a weakness of the wall of the vessel.

Anoxia. A lack of oxygen that can cause damage to cells of the brain. This can occur when blood flow to the brain is reduced.

ANP. Advanced nurse practitioner.

Anterior pelvic tilt. Forward and downward tip of the pelvis, resulting in a normal or increased lordosis of the spine.

Anticonvulsant. Medication to decrease the possibility of seizures, such as Dilantin, Trileptal, Keppra, Tegretol, Depakote, and Neurontin.

Anxiety. A feeling of apprehension, worry, uneasiness, or dread, especially of the future. Everyone has been anxious at some time. Anxiety is a normal reaction to that which threatens one's body, lifestyle, values, or loved ones. A certain amount of anxiety is normal and stimulates an individual to purposeful action. Excess anxiety interferes with the efficient functioning of an individual.

Apathy. A lack of interest or concern.

Aphasia. Impaired language or a loss of language.

Apraxia. Inability to perform purposeful movement even though the muscles are not paralyzed and the patient understands the task. This presents as a problem in planning or sequencing a desired movement, e.g., a person would not know how to get up from the floor to stand.

Aspiration. A swallowing problem when food, liquid, or secretions enter the lungs.

Ataxia. Abnormal muscle activity resulting in incoordination of movement, e.g., a person would know how to plan to get up from the floor but would perform the task with uncoordinated movement.

Attention. Ability to focus on events in the environment.

Attention span. The length of time that a person is able to focus on events in the environment.

Auditory comprehension. Understanding of spoken utterances.

Auditory tracking. The ability to locate sound.

Bed mobility. Ability to move on a mat or bed, by rolling, sitting, or lying down.

Bilateral. Both sides (of the body).

Catheter. A tube for draining urine; indwelling; inserted into the bladder (Foley) or external over the penis (condom).

Cognition. Thinking skills such as knowing, being aware, perceiving objects, remembering ideas, understanding, and reasoning.

Coma. A state of unconsciousness from which the patient cannot be aroused, even by powerful stimulation.

Concentration. Maintaining attention on a task over a period of time; remaining attentive and not easily diverted.

Concussion. Head injury resulting in the temporary loss of consciousness or the impairment of neural function.

Confabulation. Talking about people, places, and events with no basis in reality. May be delivered with apparent confidence by the individual.

Constraint therapy. A new form of therapy that focuses the person to use her unaffected limb in functional tasks while restraining the unaffected limb.

Continence. Ability to control bowel and bladder functions.

Contracture. Loss of movement at a joint secondary to muscle shortening and tightness.

Contrecoup. Bruising of brain tissue on the side opposite where the head was hit.

Contusion. A bruise of the brain resulting from a head injury.

Convergent thinking. Recognition and analysis of relevant information to identify a main theme or a main point.

Coping skills. The ability to deal with problems and difficulties by attempting to overcome them or accept them.

CT scan (computed tomography). A series of x-rays taken at different levels of the brain that depicts the brain in slices. It provides very accurate pictures of the brain.

Day care. A service provided during ordinary working hours for the patient who requires supervision, including assistance with medication, meal preparation, dressing, or moving about. However, the family returns the patient to her residence and assumes responsibility for care during the evening and at night.

Decubitus. A localized breakdown of all skin layers (commonly called a bedsore).

Deductive reasoning. Drawing conclusions based on premises or general principles in a step-by-step manner regarding a given situation.

Depression. Characterized by altered mood where there is loss of interest in all usually pleasurable activities, such as food, sex, work, friends, hobbies, leisure. There may be weight gain or loss, sleep disturbances, fatigue, feelings of worthlessness or guilt, diminished ability to think or concentrate, or recurrent thoughts of death or suicide.

Diffuse axonal injury (DAI). Damage throughout the brain to the nerve fibers that connect the nervous system.

Diffuse brain damage. Injury to cells in many different areas of the brain rather than in one specific location. Diffuse damage is common in closed-head injuries due to the brain moving about and tissue being torn, stretched, and bruised.

Discrimination. The ability to differentiate two or more stimuli.

Disorientation. Inability to report correct information regarding time, person, or place.

Divergent thinking. Generation of unique abstract concepts or hypotheses that deviate from standard concepts or ideas.

Dorsiflexion. Movement of the ankle upward toward the face.

Dysarthria. A deficit in voice and speech production caused by problems in muscle control and coordination of the lips, tongue, or throat.

Dysphagia. Impairment of oral feeding skills and swallowing.

Edema. Collection of fluid in the tissue causing swelling.

EEG (electroencephalogram). A procedure that uses electrodes on the scalp to record electrical activity of the brain.

Embolism. Obstruction of a blood vessel by foreign substances or, more frequently, a blood clot.

Emotional lability. Exhibiting rapid and drastic changes in emotional state (laughing, crying, anger) without apparent reason.

Evoked potential. An electrical response produced in a particular portion of the nervous system (e.g., spinal cord, brain stem, cerebral cortex) by stimulation of sensory receptors in the skin, the eyes, or the ears or by direct electrical stimulation of major peripheral nerves. These potentials are recorded to determine how well certain nerve circuits are functioning.

Extended-care facility. A residential facility (basically, a very skilled nursing home) for the patient who requires twenty-four-hour nursing care or rehabilitative therapy such as physical, occupational, or speech therapy on a less intensive basis than as an inpatient in a comprehensive rehabilitation center. An extended-care facility is usually a short-term alternative (two to three months) prior to placement at home (with outpatient therapy) or in a nursing home.

Fine motor control. Delicate, intricate movements as in writing or playing a piano.

Flaccid. Absence of normal muscle tension causing lack of muscle activity, e.g., limp arm or leg.

Flexion. Any bending movement of a joint.

Frustration tolerance. The ability to deal with frustrating events in daily life without becoming angry or aggressive.

Functional activity. An activity performed by a person to accomplish a useful purpose.

Gait training. Instruction in walking, with or without equipment; also called ambulation training.

Gastrostomy tube. A feeding tube passed directly into the stomach from outside the abdomen.

Glasgow coma scale. A scale used to predict the severity of a brain injury. It rates motor responses, eye opening, and verbal responses.

Gross motor control. Large, strong movements as in chopping wood or walking.

Hematoma. The collection of blood in tissues or in a space following rupture of a blood vessel.

Hemianopsia. Blindness of half the field of vision in one or both eyes.

Hemiparesis. Inability to move (paralysis of) one side of the body.

Hemorrhage. Bleeding. Cerebral: into the brain; epidural: between the skull and dura; or subdural: between the dura and brain.

ICU (Intensive Care Unit) or SCU (Special Care Unit). Hospital unit that utilizes highly sophisticated equipment and specially trained nurses to care for patients who are in such serious condition that they must be continuously monitored.

Impulsivity. The tendency to act suddenly and spontaneously without thinking of the consequences of the actions.

Independent. Ability to perform an activity consistently and safely, in a practical amount of time, without supervision or assistance.

Inflexibility. Inability to adjust to changes.

Inhibitive positioning. Those positions that interfere and break up abnormal patterns or postures of the trunk or limb caused by abnormal tone (e.g., hypertonicity).

Intracerebral. Within the tissues of the brain.

Judgment. The process of forming an opinion based on an evaluation of the situation at hand in comparison with personal values, preferences, and insights.

Lability. Loss of emotional control. This is related more to brain damage and less to depression.

Laceration. An actual tear or cut.

Learned nonuse. A theory that suggests survivors "learn" not to use an affected body part because it is more difficult.

Levels of independence. Independent, minimal assist (patient performs 75% or more of task), moderate assist (patient performs 50% to 75%), maximal assist (patient performs 25% to 50%), and dependent (patient performs less than 25%).

Long-term memory. Memory retained for an indefinite time period.

Lordosis. Natural inward or forward curve of the low back.

Medicaid. The state's program for those who need and qualify for medical assistance. It can pay for some health care services for those eligible.

Medicare. A federal health insurance program for people sixty-five or older, people of any age with permanent kidney failure, and certain people with disabilities. A person is considered disabled by Social Security when he has a severe physical or mental impairment or a combination of impairments that prevents him from working for a year or more. A person with a disability has Medicare coverage after he has received Social Security disability benefits for twenty-four months.

Memory. The process of recalling or reproducing what has been learned and retained.

Motivation. The arousal/feeling component of behavior that sees to it that a plan of action is developed and executed.

Muscle tone. The normal tension in a muscle.

Neural plasticity. The concept that the brain has the potential to "rewire" itself or utilize undamaged areas in the recovery process.

Neuropsychology. An area of psychology that relates emotions, motivations, cognition, and personality to models of brain function.

NPO. A medical abbreviation for a physician's order that the patient is to receive "nothing by mouth."

Nystagmus. Involuntary movement of the eyeball.

Orientation. Awareness of person, place, and time.

Orthosis. External support that can take the form of a brace or a splint designed to improve function or provide stability.

OT. Occupational therapy.

Outpatient. Patient living outside the hospital but requiring continuation of one or more therapies.

PA. Physician assistant.

Perception. Ability to recognize and distinguish objects in the environment, including size, shape, color, texture, smell, and sound. It is the way the brain interprets sensory information.

Perseveration. Becoming "stuck" on one word, idea, or task and not being able to switch back and forth or go on to the next word, idea, or task.

Personality. The unique organization of traits, characteristics, and modes of behavior of a person that set the person apart from others and at the same time determine how others react to the person.

Plantar flexion. Movement of the ankle downward away from the face.

Posterior pelvic tilt. Backward and upward tip of the pelvis, resulting in a flattening or decrease in the lordosis of the spine.

Pragmatics. Practical use of speech and language in a conversational setting.

Premorbid. A term to describe the patient's condition before the injury.

Primitive reflexes. Involuntary responses/reflexes present in all newborn infants that disappear in normal infants as the child's brain develops and more conscious voluntary responses emerge. These reflexes may reappear after a traumatic brain injury.

Problem-solving skills. Ability to consider the probable factors that can influence the outcome of each of various solutions to a problem and to select the most advantageous solution. Patients with deficits in these skills may become "immobilized" when faced with a problem. Because they are unable to think of possible solutions, they respond by doing nothing.

Prognosis. The prospect as to recovery from a disease or injury as indicated by the nature and symptoms of the case.

Prone. A position of lying on one's stomach.

Proprioception. The sense of knowing where one's limb is in space statically once the limb has stopped moving.

Prosthesis. An artificial limb.

PTA (post-traumatic amnesia). The period of time after an injury when the patient suffers a loss of day-to-day memory. The patient is unable to store new information and, therefore, has a decreased ability to learn. Memory of the PTA period is never stored; therefore, things that happened during that period cannot be recalled.

Quadriplegia. Paralysis involving both legs and both arms.

Recall. The ability to remember (immediate and delayed recall).

Reflex. Unconscious involuntary movement in response to a stimulus.

Rehabilitation. A system of organized treatment that enables an injured patient to regain the highest possible level of mental and physical ability.

ROM (range of motion). Taking a joint through the available range. This movement may be passive (someone other than the patient moves the limb), active assistance (the patient tries moving the limb as far as possible and then someone else takes the limb to the end of the available range), or active (the patient moves the limb independent of any help).

Rote memory. Storage and retrieval of information without comprehension.

Seizures. Episodes of altered consciousness that may be associated with jerking movements resulting from abnormal electrical activity in the brain.

Selective attention. Ability to select discrete elements of environment and block out extraneous stimuli.

Sensory stimulation. The process of providing input to the senses—touch, smell, sight, taste, hearing. Sensory stimulation provides something for the patient to respond to. A response is the beginning of the process toward meaningful activity.

Serial casting. Use of a series of casts around a joint to stretch contractures and increase the range of motion in a joint.

Short-term memory. Memory retained for only a relatively brief period of time.

Social Security Disability Insurance (SSDI). Eligibility is based on: (1) a person having a severe physical or mental impairment or a combination of both that prevents him or her from working for a year or more and (2) a person having worked long enough and recently enough under Social Security to be insured.

Spasticity. Imbalance of muscle tension causing resistance to passive motion, e.g., if one tries to bend or straighten the elbows, the muscles on one side of the joint resist the movement.

Spontaneous recovery. The recovery that occurs as damage to body tissue heals. This type of recovery occurs with or without rehabilitation and it's very difficult to know how much improvement is spontaneous and how much is due to rehabilitative interventions. However, when the recovery is guided by an experienced rehabilitation team, complications can be anticipated and minimized; the return of function can be channeled in useful directions and in progressive steps so that the eventual outcome is the best that is possible.

Stimulus. Agent, act, or influence that produces a reaction.

Subdural. Beneath the dura (tough membrane covering the brain and spinal cord).

Supine. A position of lying on one's back.

Supplemental Security Income (SSI). Federal program run by Social Security that pays monthly checks to people who are aged, blind, or disabled and have very limited income and financial resources. Eligibility is based on: (1) a person having a physical or mental disability that is expected to keep him or her from working for at least twelve months; (2) an individual's total monthly income and financial resources, e.g., savings, checking accounts, bonds, CDs, property, and cash-value life insurance. Individuals eligible for SSI receive Medicaid.

Tangentiality. The surface structure of language output appears to be intact; however, conceptual confusion is obvious and is reflected in problems of poor word selection, loose connection of thoughts and ideas, impairment in abstract thinking, and a strong tendency to stray from the core of the message or topic.

Thrombosis. The formation, development, or existence of a blood clot within the vascular system. The clot can occlude a vessel and stop the blood supply to the brain or other organ. If the thrombus detaches, it becomes an embolus and may occlude a vessel at a distance from the original site.

Trach; Tracheostomy. A surgical opening at the front of the throat providing access to the trachea or windpipe.

Transfer. Refers to methods of getting to and from a wheelchair, bed, toilet, etc., using a stand-pivot movement or a sliding board, for example.

Unilateral neglect. Ignoring items on one side of the body.

Ventricles. Four natural cavities in the brain that are filled with cerebrospinal fluid.

Vestibular. Pertaining to the vestibular system in the middle ear and the brain that senses movement of the head. Disorders of the vestibular system can lead to dizziness, poor regulation of postural muscle tone, and inability to detect quick movements of the head.

Visual tracking. The ability to follow an object, person, or light up, down, and to the left and right.

Void. To urinate or defecate.

Word-finding problem. Decreased ability to retrieve words, much like "tip-of-the-tongue" syndrome.

Sources

Albert, M. L., MD, D. L. Bachman, MD, A. Morgan, PhD, and N. Helm-Estabrooks, ScD, "Pharmacotherapy for Aphasia," *Neurology* 38 (June 1988).

Albert, M. L., MD, and N. Helm-Estabrooks, "Diagnosis and Treatment of Aphasia: Part I," *Journal of the American Medical Association* 259: 7 (February 19, 1988).

Anderson, T. P., "Rehabilitation of Patients with Completed Stroke," in *Krusen's Handbook of Physical Medicine and Rehabilitation, 4th Edition,* Ed. by F. Kottke and J. F. Lehmann (Philadelphia: W. B. Saunders, 1990).

Bach-y-Rita, P., "Brain Plasticity as a Basis of the Development of Rehabilitation Procedures for Hemiplegia," *Scandinavian Journal of Rehabilitation Medicine* 13 (1981).

Barnett, H. J. M., MD, "The Contribution of Multicenter Trials to Stroke Prevention and Treatment," *Archives of Neurology* 47 (April 1990).

Beck, A. T., R. A. Steer, and M. G. Garbin, "Psychometric Properties of the Beck Depression Inventory: Twenty-Five Years of Evaluation," *Clinical Psychology Review* 8(1), 77–100 (1988).

Beck, A. T., C. H. Ward, M. Mendelson, J. Mock, and J. Erbaugh, "An Inventory for Measuring Depression," *Archives of General Psychiatry* 4: 561–71 (1961).

Bishop, D. S., MD, and R. L. Evans, ACSW, "Family Functioning Assessment Techniques in Stroke," *Stroke, Supplement II* 21 (1990).

Bleiberg, J., PhD, "Psychological and Neuropsychological Factors in Stroke Management," in *Stroke Rehabilitation,* Ed. by P. E. Kaplan, MD, and L. J. Cerullo, MD (Boston: Butterworth, 1986).

Boston Diagnostic Aphasia Examination (BDAE).

Brodal, A., "Self-Observations and Neuro-Anatomical Considerations After a Stroke," *Brain* 96 (1973).

Brody, J., "What Is a Stroke," *Be Stroke Smart* paper (Englewood, CO: National Stroke Association).

Burns, M. S., PhD, "Language Without Communication: The Pragmatics of Right Hemisphere Damage," in *Clinical Management of Right Hemisphere Dysfunction,* Ed. by M. S. Burns, A. S. Halper, and S. I. Mogil (Rockville, MD: Aspen Publishers, 1985).

Caplan, L. R., MD, "Stroke," *Clinical Symposia* 40: 4 (Summit, NJ: CIBA-GEIGY, 1988).

Charness, A., MS, "Stroke/Head Injury: A Guide to Functional Outcomes," in *Physical Therapy Management* (Rockville, MD: Aspen Publishers, 1986).

Coughlan, A. K., "The Wimbledon Self-Report Scale: Emotional and Mood Appraisal," *Clinical Rehabilitation* 2 (1988).

Craig, C., "Household Barriers Confronting the Stroke Survivor," *Be Stroke Smart* paper (Englewood, CO: National Stroke Association).

Cummings, J. L., MD, "Neurological Syndromes Associated with Right Hemisphere Damage," in *Clinical Management of Right Hemisphere Dysfunction,* Ed. by M. S. Burns, A. S. Halper, and S. I. Mogil (Rockville, MD: Aspen Publishers, 1985).

Dawson, T. C., MSW, "Depression: A Natural Reaction to Stroke," *Be Stroke Smart* paper (Englewood, CO: National Stroke Association).

DeJong, G., and L. G. Branch, "Predicting the Stroke Patient's Ability to Live Independently," *Stroke* 13 (1982).

Dobkin, B. H., "Rehabilitation After Stroke," *New England Journal of Medicine* 352: 1677–84 (2005).

Dombovy, M. L., Basford, J. R., et al., "Disability and Use of Rehabilitation Services Following Stroke in Rochester, Minnesota," *Stroke* 18: 830–36 (1987).

Dumont, L., MD, *Surviving Adolescence* (New York: Villard Books, 1991).

Duncan, P. W., R. D. Horner, et al., "Adherence to Post Acute Rehabilitation Guidelines Is Associated with Functional Recovery in Stroke," *Stroke* 33: 167–78 (2002).

Entwistle, B., "Dental Health Care for the Stroke Survivor," *Be Stroke Smart* paper (Englewood, CO: National Stroke Association).

Evans, R. L., ACSW, and D. S. Bishop, MD, "Psychosocial Outcomes in Stroke Survivors," *Stroke, Supplement II* 21 (1990).

Farrar, J., "Aphasia: Prison Without Walls," *Be Stroke Smart* paper (Englewood, CO: National Stroke Association).

Fedoroff, J. P., MD, and R. G. Robinson, MD, "Tricyclic Antidepressants in the Treatment of Poststroke Depression," *Journal of Clinical Psychiatry* 50: 7 (July 1989).

Finklestein, S., MD, L. I. Benowitz, PhD, R. J. Baldessarini, MD, G. W. Arana, MD, D. Levine, MD, E. Woo, MD, D. Bear, MD, K. Moya, BA, and A. L. Stoll, BA, "Mood, Vegetative Disturbance, and Dexamethasone Suppression Test After Stroke," *Annals of Neurology* 12 (1982).

Forrester, L.V., L. A. Wheaten, and A. R. Luft, "Exercise-Mediated Locomotor Recovery and Lower-Limb Neuroplasticity After Stroke," *Journal of Rehabilitation Research and Development* 45 (2008).

Frumkin, N. L., E. J. Potchen, A. S. Aniskiewicz, J. B. Moore, and P. A. Cooke, "Potential Impact of Magnetic Resonance Imaging on the Field of Communication Disorders," *ASHA* (August 1989).

Garrison, S. J., L. A. Rolak, R. R. Dodaro, and A. J. O'Callaghan, "Rehabilitation of the Stroke Patient," in *Rehabilitation Medicine: Principles and Practice,* Ed. by J. DeLisa (New York: J. B. Lippincott, 1988).

Gold, P. W., MD, F. K. Goodwin, MD, and G. P. Chrousos, MD, "Clinical and Biochemical Manifestations of Depression:

Relation to the Neurobiology of Stress, First of Two Parts," *New England Journal of Medicine* 319: 6 (August 11, 1988).

Gold, P. W., MD, F. K. Goodwin, MD, and G. P. Chrousos, MD, "Clinical and Biochemical Manifestations of Depression: Relation to the Neurobiology of Stress, Second of Two Parts," *New England Journal of Medicine* 319: 7 (August 18, 1988).

Granger, C. V., MD, L. S. Dewis, MD, N. C. Peters, MEd, C. C. Sherwood, PhD, and J. E. Barrett, BA, "Stroke Rehabilitation: Analysis of Repeated Barthel Index Measures," *Archives of Physical Medicine Rehabilitation* 60 (January 1979).

Greenwood, J., MEd, "A Practical Approach to Swallowing Disorders: Part II," *Progress Report, A Rehabilitation Journal* 3: 1 (1990).

Greenwood, J., MEd, and R. C. Senelick, MD, "A Practical Approach to Swallowing Disorders: Part I," *Progress Report, A Rehabilitation Journal* 3: 1 (1990).

Hachinksi, V., MD, "Brain Attacks," *Be Stroke Smart* 7: 3 (Winter 1990).

Hachinksi, V., MD, "Classification of Stroke for Clinical Trials," *Stroke, Supplement II* 21: 9 (1990).

Hagen, C., PhD, "Communication Abilities in Hemiplegia: Effect of Speech in Therapy," *Archives of Physical Medicine and Rehabilitation* 54 (October 1973).

Halper, A. S., MA, and S. I. Mogil, MS, "Communication Disorders: Diagnosis and Treatment," in *Stroke Rehabilitation*, Ed. by P. E. Kaplan, MD, and L. J. Cerullo, MD (Boston: Butterworth, 1986).

Herbert, P. R., J. M. Gaziano, K. S. Chan, and C. H. Hennekens, "Cholesterol Lowering with Statin Drugs, Risk of Stroke, and Total Mortality: An Overview of Randomized Trials," *Journal of the American Medical Association* 278 (1997).

Hershey, L. A., MD, PhD, "Dementia Associated With Stroke," *Stroke,* Supplement II 21 (1990).

Hertanu, J. S., MD, J. T. Demopoulos, MD, W. C. Yang, MD, W. F. Calhoun, PhD, and H. A. Fenigstein, OTR, "Stroke Rehabilitation: Correlation and Prognostic Value of Computerized Tomography and Sequential Functional Assessments," *Archives of Physical Medicine Rehabilitation* 65 (September 1984).

Hesson, L. F., "Use of Braces to Help Regain Control of the Foot/ Ankle," *Be Stroke Smart* paper (Englewood, CO: National Stroke Association).

Hier, D. B., MD, J. Mondlock, and L. R. Caplan, "Recovery of Behavorial Abnormalities After Right Hemisphere Stroke," *Neurology* (March 1983).

Hilts, P. J., "A Brain Unit Seen as Index for Recalling Memories," *The New York Times* (September 24, 1991).

"Hypertension and Diabetes," *National Stroke Association Newsletter* 6: 4 (Winter 1989).

Jongbloed, L., "Prediction of Function After Stroke: A Critical Review," *Stroke* 17 (1986).

Jorgensen, H. S., H. Nakayama, et al., "Outcome and Time Course of Recovery in Stroke. Part I: Outcome. The Copenhagen Stroke Study," *Archives of Physical Medicine Rehabilitation* 76 (1995).

Kaplan, P. E., "Hemiplegia: Rehabilitation of the Lower Extremity," in *Stroke Rehabilitation,* Ed. by P. E. Kaplan, MD, and L. J. Cerullo, MD (Boston: Butterworth, 1986).

Kelly-Hayes, M., EdD, "Time Intervals, Survival, and Destination: Three Crucial Variables in Stroke Outcome Research," *Stroke, Supplement II* 21: 9 (September 1990).

Kemperman, G., H. G. Kahn, and F. H. Gage, "More Hippocampal Neurons in Adult Mice Living in Enriched Environment," *Nature* 386: 493–95 (1997).

Kemperman, G., H. van Pragg, and F. H. Gage, "Activity Dependent Regulation of Neuronal Plasticity and Self Repair," *Prog Brain Res* 127: 35–48 (2000).

Kozy, M. C., and G. A. Tarvin, "Working with Families," in *Clinical Management of Right Hemisphere Dysfunction,* Ed. by M. S. Burns, A. S. Halper, and S. T. Mogil, p. 98 (Rockville, MD: Aspen Publishers, 1985).

Kramer, A. M., J. C. Kowalsky, et al., "Outcome and Utilization Differences for Older Persons with Stroke in HMO and Fee for Service Systems," *JAGS* 48: 726–34 (2000).

Kramer, A. M., R. E. Schlenker, et al., "Stroke Rehabilitation in Nursing Homes," *Top Stroke Rehabilitation* 4: 53–63 (1997).

Langhorne, P., and L. Legg, "Evidence Behind Stroke Rehabilitation," *J Neurol Neurosurg Psychiatry, Supplement* IV 73: 18–21 (2003).

Lavin, J. H., "There Is Sex After Stroke," *Be Stroke Smart* paper (Englewood, CO: National Stroke Association).

Lavin, J. H., "What Every Family Should Know About Stroke," *Be Stroke Smart* paper (Englewood, CO: National Stroke Association).

Leary, W. E., "Older People Enjoy Sex, Survey Says," *The New York Times* (September 29, 1998).

Lehmann, J. F., B. J. DeLateur, et al., "Stroke. Does Rehabilitation Affect Outcome?" *Archives of Physical Medicine Rehabilitation* 56 (1975).

Lieberman, J. S., MD, "Hemiplegia: Rehabilitation of the Upper Extremity," in *Stroke Rehabilitation,* Ed. by P. E. Kaplan, MD, and L. J. Cerullo, MD (Boston: Butterworth, 1986).

Lindmark, B., "The Improvement of Different Motor Functions After Stroke," *Clinical Rehabilitation* 2 (1988).

Lipsey, J. R., R. G. Robinson, G. D. Pearlson, K. Rao, and T. R. Price, "Nortriptyline Treatment of Post-Stroke Depression: A Double-Blind Study," *The Lancet* (February 11, 1984).

McDowell, F., MD, and S. Louis, MD, "Improvement in Motor Performance in Paretic and Paralyzed Extremities Following Nonembolic Cerebral Infarction," *Stroke* 2 (July–August 1971).

Meeks, J. E., MD, *High Time/Low Times: How to Cope with Teenage Depression* (New York: Berkley Books, 1989).

Millikan, C. H., MD, F. McDowell, MD, and J. D. Easton, MD, *Stroke* (Philadelphia: Lea & Febiger, 1987).

Moskowitz, E., MD, F. E. H. Lightbody, MD, and N. S. Freitag, RN, "Long-Term Follow-Up of the Poststroke Patient," *Archives of Physical Medicine and Rehabilitation* (April 1972).

NINDS Stroke Study Group, "Tissue Plasminogen Activator for Acute Ischemic Stroke," *New England Journal of Medicine* 333: 1581–87 (1995).

North American Symptomatic Carotid Endarterectomy Trial Collaborators, "Beneficial Effect of Carotid Endarterectomy in Symptomatic Patients with High-Grade Carotid Stenosis," *New England Journal of Medicine* 525: 445–53 (1991).

Novak, T. A., MA, W. T. Satterfield, K. Lyons et al., "Stroke Onset and Rehabilitation: Time Lag as a Factor in Treatment Outcome," *Archives of Physical Medicine and Rehabilitation* 65 (June 1984).

Nudo, R. J., "Recovery after Damage to Motor Corical Areas," *Current Opinions in Neurobiology* 9: 740–47 (1999).

Nudo, R. J., "Remodeling of Corical Motor Representations After Stroke: Implications for Recovery from Brain Damage," *Molecular Psychiatry* 2: 188–91 (1997).

Nudo, R. J., and G. W. Milliken, "Reorganization of Movement Representations in Primary Motor Cortex Following Ischemic Infarcts in Squirrel Monkeys," *Journal of Neurophysiology* 75: 2144–49 (1996).

Nudo, R. J., E. J. Plautz, and G. H. Milliken, "Adaptive Plasticity in Primate Motor Cortex as a Consequence of Behavioral Experience and Neuronal Injury," *Seminars in Neuroscience* 9: 13–23 (1997).

Nursing Homes Outcome Initiative (Rand DRU-2863, September 2002).

Olson, D. A., PhD, "Management of Non-Language Behavior in the Stroke Patient," in *Stroke Rehabilitation,* Ed. by P. E.

Kaplan, MD, and L. J. Cerullo, MD (Boston: Butterworth, 1986).

Papanicolaou, A. C., PhD, B. D. Moore, PhD, G. Deutsch, PhD, H. S. Levin, PhD, and H. M. Eisenberg, MD, "Evidence for Right-Hemisphere Involvement in Recovery from Aphasia," *Archives of Neurology* 45 (September 1988).

Partridge, C. J., M. Johnston, and S. Edwards, "Recovery from Physical Disability after Stroke: Normal Patterns as a Basis for Evaluation," *The Lancet* (February 14, 1987).

Pfalzgraf, B., MA, "Coping with Stroke and Aphasia as a Family," *Be Stroke Smart* 7: 3 (Winter 1990).

"Positioning the Stroke Survivor with Paralysis," *Be Stroke Smart* paper (Englewood, CO: National Stroke Association).

Price, T. R., MD, "Affective Disorders After Stroke," *Stroke, Supplement II* 21 (1990).

Quizilbash, N., S. W. Duffy, C. Warlow, and I. Mann, "Lipids Are Risk Factors for Ischemic Stroke: Overview and Review," *Cerebrovascular Disease* 2 (1992).

"Recognition and Management of Post-Stroke Depression," *Stroke Clinical Updates II,* 1 (May 1991).

Retchin, S. M., MD, R. S. Brown, PhD, S. J. Yeh, MS, D. Chu, and L. Moreno, PhD, "Outcomes of Stroke Patients in Medicare Fee for Service and Managed Care," *Journal of the American Medical Association* 278: 2 (July 9, 1997).

Rippe, J. M., MD, and A. Ward, PhD, with K. Dougherty, *The Rockport Walking Program* (New York: Prentice Hall, 1989).

Rosenberg, S. J., MD, and J. J. Fadem, MD, "Geriatric Neurology: Five Acute Problems," *Emergency Medicine* (September 30, 1992).

Rossi, P. W., "Stroke," in *Orthotics in Neurological Rehabilitation,* Ed. by M. L. Aisen, MD (New York: Demos Publications, 1992).

Sacco, R. L., E . J. Benjamin, J. P. Broderick, et al., "Risk Factors: Panel—American Heart Association Prevention Conference IV," *Stroke* 28 (1997).

Sacco, R. L., BS, P. A. Wolf, MD, W. B. Kannel, MD, and P. M. McNamara, "Survival and Recurrence Following Stroke: The Framingham Study," *Stroke* 13: 3 (May–June 1982).

Schaefer, S., "Bladder Problems Following Stroke," *Be Stroke Smart* paper (Englewood, CO: National Stroke Association).

Schmidt, J. G., J. Drew-Cates, and M. L. Dombovy, "Severe Disability After Stroke: Outcome After Inpatient Rehabilitation," *Neurorehabilitation and Neural Repair* 13: 199–203 (1999).

"Self-Help Devices for the Kitchen," *Be Stroke Smart* paper (Englewood, CO: National Stroke Association).

Senelick, R. C., "The Other Side: Disorders of the Right Hemisphere," *Progress Report, A Rehabilitation Journal* 3: 3 (1991).

Senelick, R. C., MD, and C. E. Ryan, *Living with Head Injury* (Washington, DC: RHSC Press, 1991).

Shah, S., F. Vanclay, et al., "Predicting Discharge Status at Commencement of Stroke Rehabilitation," *Stroke* 20: 766–69 (1989).

SHEP Cooperative Research Group, "Prevention of Stroke by Antihypertensive Drug Treatment in Older Persons with Isolated Systolic Hypertension: Final Results of the Systolic Hypertension in the Elderly Program (SHEP)," *Journal of the American Medication Association* 265 (1991).

Shewan, C. M., "The Language Quotient (LQ): A New Measure for the Western Aphasia Battery," *Journal of Communication Disorders* 19 (1986).

Skilled Nursing Facilities: Providers Have Responded to Medicare Payment System by Changing Practices (GAO-02-841, August 2002).

Slaby, A., MD, PhD, *Aftershock: Surviving the Delayed Effects of Traumas, Crisis, and Loss* (New York: Villard Books, 1989).

Staessen, J. A., R. Fagard, L. Thijs, et al., "Syst-Eur Trial Investigators: Randomised Double-Blind Comparison of Placebo and Active Treatment for Older Patients with Isolated Systolic Hypertension," *The Lancet* 350 (1997).

Stern, P. H., MD, F. McDowell, MD, J. M. Miller, PhD, and M. Robinson, RN, "Factors Influencing Stroke Rehabilitation," *Stroke* 2 (May–June 1971).

"Stroke Clubs," *Be Stroke Smart* paper (Englewood, CO: National Stroke Association).

"Stroke in the Young—Cardiac Causes," *Stroke Clinical Updates* 1: 4 (November 1990).

"Stroke in the Young Patient—Coagulation Disturbances," *Stroke Clinical Updates* 1 (September 1990).

"Stroke Prevention: The Importance of Risk Factors," *Stroke Clinical Updates* 1: 5 (January 1991).

"The Stroke Support Group," *Be Stroke Smart* paper (Englewood, CO: National Stroke Association).

Tampa General Rehabilitation Center, *Actions and Reactions: A Stroke Manual for Families* (Houston, TX: HDI Publishers, 1989).

Taub, E., N. E. Miller, et al., "Technique to Improve Chronic Motor Deficit After Stroke," *Archives of Physical Medical Rehabilitation* 74: 347–54 (1993).

"Therapeutic Recreation," *Be Stroke Smart* paper (Englewood, CO: National Stroke Association).

Understanding Stroke Rehabilitation (Allentown, PA: Good Shepherd Rehabilitation Hospital, 1988).

Vanclay, F., "Functional Outcome Measures in Stroke Rehabilitation," *Stroke* 22: 105–108 (1991).

Wade, D. T., MD, and R. L. Hewer, MD, "Stroke: Associations with Age, Sex, and Side of Weakness," *Archives of Physical Medical Rehabilitation* 67 (August 1986).

Wardlaw, J. M., C. P. Warlow, and C. Counsell, "Systematic Review of Evidence on Thrombolytic Therapy for Acute Ischaemic Stroke," *The Lancet* 350 (1997).

Wender, D., PhD, "Aphasic Victim as Investigator," *Archives of Neurology* 46 (January 1989).

Wertz, R. T., PhD, "Communication Deficits in Stroke Survivors: An Overview of Classification and Treatment," *Stroke, Supplement II* 21 (1990).

Wolf, P. A., R. D. Abbott, and W. B. Kannel, "Atrial Fibrillation as an Independent Risk Factor for Stroke: The Framingham Study," *Stroke* 22 (1991).

Wolf, S. L., PhD, "Use of Biofeedback in the Treatment of Stroke Patients," *Stroke, Supplement II* 21 (1990).

Wolf, S. L., D. E. LeCraw, et al., "Forced Use of Hemiplegic Upper Extremities to Reverse the Effect of Learned Nonuse Among Chronic Stroke and Head-Injured Patients," *Experimental Neurology* 104: 125–32 (1989).

Zubenko, G. S., MD, PhD, and J. Mossey, MD, "Major Depression in Primary Dementia: Clinical and Neuropathologic Correlates," *Archives of Neurology* 45 (November 1988).

Index

About the Author

Richard C. Senelick, M.D., is a physician specializing in both neurology and the subspecialty of neurorehabilitation. He is the editor-in-chief of Encompass Health Press. Dr. Senelick served as the medical director of HealthSouth Rehabilitation Institute of San Antonio (RIOSA) for 30 years. He is the professor in the department of neurology at the University of Texas Health Science Center in San Antonio. Dr. Senelick writes a blog on healthcare-related issues for the Huffington Post and The Atlantic. In addition, Dr. Senelick is the stroke community expert for WebMD, the largest source of online health information. He is a frequently sought-after speaker both nationally and internationally. Amongst his many books and publications, he has authored "Living with Brain Injury: A Guide for Patients and Their Families," "The Spinal Cord Injury Handbook" and "Multiple Sclerosis: The New Journey."